W9-CPF-889

Mini Medications and Mothers' Milk 2010
Fourteenth Edition

Thomas W. Hale, R.Ph., Ph.D.
Professor of Pediatrics
Associate Dean of Research
Texas Tech University
School of Medicine
Amarillo, Texas 79106

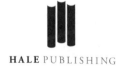

HALE PUBLISHING

1712 N. Forest St. Amarillo, Texas 79106

Mini Medications and Mothers' Milk 2010
Fourteenth Edition

Hale Publishing, L.P.

1712 N. Forest St.

Amarillo, TX 79106-7017

www.iBreastfeeding.com

(806)-376-9900

(800)-378-1317

DISCLAIMER

ISBN13: 978-0-9845039-5-7

Library of Congress Number: 2010938252

Printing and Binding: Malloy
Cover Printing: Malloy

Printed in the USA

Preface

Many healthcare providers have told us that it would be ideal if they had a copy of *Medications and Mothers' Milk* available at all times. With so many medications on the market, for so many conditions, it can be difficult to keep track of which ones are safest for breastfeeding women. Working at a medical school, I see medical students and residents who are usually on the move, working with patients in a variety of settings, often far away from their reference materials. These same physicians in training often make use of smaller versions of their favorite references that they can easily slip into their pockets and carry with them as they see patients. Clinicians can also use pocket versions of their favorite references as they work in a variety of home and office settings.

It was with these needs in mind that we have produced the miniature version of *Medications and Mothers' Milk*—also known as "*Mini-Meds*." In this book, we have tried to distill the body of knowledge on lactational pharmacology into its smallest format so that it will be within reach of lactation specialists' coat pockets.

The purpose of *Mini-Meds* is to provide on-the-spot information about medications that can be used at bedside, but with less detail than the full edition. It is not meant to stand on its own as a text. As such, *Mini-Meds* is not meant to be a replacement for the full edition of *Medications and Mothers' Milk*. Rather, it is a quick reminder, and the full text can be consulted as time permits. Therefore, *Mini-Meds* and *Medications and Mothers' Milk* are companion volumes; complementary, but not interchangeable. We hope you will find this useful in your work.

Thomas W. Hale, Ph.D.

How To Use This Book

This section of the book is designed to aid the reader in determining risk to an infant from maternal medications and in using the pharmacokinetic parameters throughout this reference.

Drug Description and Kinetics

Drug Name and Generic Name
Each monograph begins with the generic name of the drug. Several of the most common USA trade names are provided under the Trade section.

Uses
This lists the general use of the medication, such as penicillin antibiotic, or antiemetic, or analgesic, etc. Remember, many drugs have multiple uses in many syndromes. I have only listed the most common use.

AAP
This entry lists the new recommendations provided by the American Academy of Pediatrics as published in their document, The transfer of drugs and other chemicals into human milk (Pediatrics. 2001 Sep;108(3):776-89.) Drugs are listed in tables according to the following recommendations: Cytotoxic drugs that may interfere with cellular metabolism of the nursing infant; Drugs of abuse for which adverse effects on the infant during breastfeeding have been reported; Radioactive compounds that require temporary cessation of breastfeeding; Drugs for which the effect on nursing infants is unknown but may be of concern; Drugs that have been associated with significant effects on some nursing infants and should be given to nursing mothers with caution; Maternal medication usually compatible with breastfeeding. In this book, the AAP recommendations have been paraphrased to reflect these recommendations. Because the AAP recommendations do not cover all drugs, "Not Reviewed" simply implies that the drug has not yet been reviewed by this committee. The author recommends that each user review these recommendations for further detail.

Relative Infant Dose
The relative infant dose (RID) is calculated by dividing the infants dose via milk (Theoretic Infant Dose) in "mg/kg/day" by the maternal dose in "mg/kg/day." This weight-normalizing method gives one a feeling for just how much of the "maternal dose" the infant is receiving. Most who work in this field suggest that anything less than 10% of the maternal dose is probably safe.

T½ =
This lists the most commonly recorded adult half-life of the medication.

Oral=
Oral bioavailability refers to the ability of a drug to reach the systemic circulation after oral administration. It is generally a good indication of the amount of medication that is absorbed into the blood stream of the patient. Drugs with low oral bioavailability are generally either poorly absorbed in the gastrointestinal tract, are destroyed in the gut, or are sequestered by the liver prior to entering the plasma compartment.

MW=
The molecular weight of a medication is a significant determinant as to the entry of that medication into human milk. Medications with small molecular weights (< 200) can easily pass into milk by traversing small pores in the cell walls of the mammary epithelium (see ethanol). Drugs with higher molecular weights must traverse the membrane by dissolving in the cells' lipid membranes, which may significantly reduce milk levels.

Pregnancy Risk Categories

Pregnancy risk categories have been assigned to almost all medications by their manufacturers and are based on the level of risk the drug poses to the fetus during gestation. They are not useful in assigning risk via breastfeeding. The FDA has provided these five categories to indicate the risk associated with the induction of birth defects. Unfortunately, they do not indicate the importance of when during gestation the medication is used. For this reason, I have added small comments to indicate that some drugs are more dangerous during certain trimesters of pregnancy. The definitions provided below are, however, a useful tool in determining the possible risks associated with using the medication during pregnancy. Some newer medications may not yet have pregnancy classifications and are therefore not provided herein.

Category A
Controlled studies in women fail to demonstrate a risk to the fetus in the first trimester (and there is no evidence of a risk in later trimesters) and the possibility of fetal harm appears remote.

Category B
Either animal-reproduction studies have not demonstrated a fetal risk, but there are no controlled studies in pregnant women, or animal-reproduction studies have shown an adverse effect (other than a decrease in fertility) that was not confirmed in controlled studies in women in the first trimester (and there is no evidence of a risk in later trimesters).

Category C
Either studies in animals have revealed adverse effects on the fetus (teratogenic or embryocidal, or other) and there are no controlled studies in women, or studies in women and animals are not available. Drugs should be given only if the potential benefit justifies the potential risk to the fetus.

Category D
There is positive evidence of human fetal risk, but the benefits from use in pregnant women may be acceptable despite the risk (e.g., if the drug is needed in a life-threatening situation or for a serious disease for which safer drugs cannot be used or are ineffective).

Category X
Studies in animals or human beings have demonstrated fetal abnormalities, or there is evidence of fetal risk based on human experience, or both, and the risk of the use of the drug in pregnant women clearly outweighs any possible benefit. The drug is contraindicated in women who are or may become pregnant.

Dr. Hale's Lactation Risk Categories

L1   SAFEST

Drug which has been taken by a large number of breastfeeding mothers without any observed increase in adverse effects in the infant. Controlled studies in breastfeeding women fail to demonstrate a risk to the infant and the possibility of harm to the breastfeeding infant is remote; or the product is not orally bioavailable in an infant.

L2   SAFER

Drug which has been studied in a limited number of breastfeeding women without an increase in adverse effects in the infant. And/or, the evidence of a demonstrated risk which is likely to follow use of this medication in a breastfeeding woman is remote.

L3   MODERATELY SAFE

There are no controlled studies in breastfeeding women, however, the risk of untoward effects to a breastfed infant is possible; or, controlled studies show only minimal non-threatening adverse effects. Drugs should be given only if the potential benefit justifies the potential risk to the infant. (New medications that have absolutely no published data are automatically categorized in this category, regardless of how safe they may be.)

L4   POSSIBLY HAZARDOUS

There is positive evidence of risk to a breastfed infant or to breastmilk production, but the benefits from use in breastfeeding mothers may be acceptable despite the risk to the infant (e.g., if the drug is needed in a life-threatening situation or for a serious disease for which safer drugs cannot be used or are ineffective.)

L5   CONTRAINDICATED

Studies in breastfeeding mothers have demonstrated that there is significant and documented risk to the infant based on human experience, or it is a medication that has a high risk of causing significant damage to an infant. The risk of using the drug in breastfeeding women clearly outweighs any possible benefit from breastfeeding. The drug is contraindicated in women who are breastfeeding an infant.

^{11}C-WAY 100635 or ^{11}C-RACLOPRIDE; *C-Way 100635, C-Raclopride* — L2

Uses: Diagnostic Agent, Radiopharmaceutical Imaging

AAP: Not reviewed

$T\frac{1}{2}$= 20.3 minutes;   **RID=** ;   **Oral** = ;   **MW=**

Clinical: This is a short half-life radioactive product (20.3 minutes). A brief interruption of only 100 minutes would prevent most transfer. While the radioactivity was present in milk, the tracers themselves were undetectable in the milk compartment after 90 or more minutes.

5-HYDROXYTRYPTOPHAN; *PowerSleep, Oxitriptan* — L3

Uses: Precursor of serotonin

AAP: Advise not to breastfeed

$T\frac{1}{2}$= 4.3 hours;   **RID=** ;   **Oral** = <70%;   **MW=** 393

Clinical: 5-hydroxytroptophan is likely excreted into human milk since it easily passes through the blood brain barrier. The effects toward the infant are unknown, use during breastfeeding is ill advised. Usage of L-Tryptophan for depression is not recommended due to the extremely high doses needed and lack of effectiveness. Suitable alternatives for depressions are the SSRIs and tricyclic antidepressants.

^{99m}TECHNETIUM TC SESTAMIBI; *Cardiolite, Sestamibi* — L4

Uses: Imaging agent   C

AAP: Radioactive compound that requires temporary cessation of breastfeeding

$T\frac{1}{2}$= 6 hours;   **RID=** ;   **Oral** = Complete;   **MW=**

Clinical: Technetium ^{99m} sestamibi administration may present some risk for a short-time period. Transfer to milk is unlikely since it tends to bind preferentially and irreversibly to myocardial tissue. The half-life is 6 hours, and so pumping and dumping for a day may be advised. Normal breastfeeding may be resumed afterwards.

ABACAVIR

Uses: Antiretroviral agent   C

AAP: Not reviewed

T½= ; **RID=** ; **Oral =** ; **MW=**

Clinical: Continued administration of abacavir used in combination with other antiretrovirals in an HIV patient is advised. However, HIV patients should not breastfeed since there is a high risk of transmission of the virus to the infant.

ABATACEPT; *Orencia*	L3
Uses: Antirheumatic	C

AAP: Not reviewed

T½= 13.1 days; **RID=** ; **Oral =** Nil; **MW=** 92,000

Clinical: The molecular weight of abatacept is 92 kilodaltons, extremely high. The likelihood of such a large molecule passing into milk is minimal. We have obtained no data on its transfer into milk. Administration of abatacept is probably okay. High risk of infections when taking abatacept.

ACAMPROSATE; *Campral*	L3
Uses: GABA Agonist / Glutamate Antagonist	C

AAP: Not reviewed

T½= 20-33 hours; **RID=** ; **Oral =** 11%; **MW=** 400

Clinical: The transfer into milk when published will probably be low, and its oral bioavailability is low. Further, it has a huge volume of distribution which would reduce milk levels. However, breastfeeding in alcoholic mothers is not necessarily a good idea and the relative low risk of this drug should be evaluated with the relative high risk of chronic alcohol consumption by the mother.

ACARBOSE; *Precose, Prandase, Glucobay*	L3
Uses: Delays carbohydrate absorption	B

AAP: Not reviewed

T½= <2 hours; **RID=** ; **Oral =** 0.7- 2%; **MW=** 645

Clinical: The oral bioavailability of acarbose is relatively low (2%). Thus, it is highly unlikely that acarbose would enter human milk in clinically relevant concentrations. The adverse effects are mild and mainly gastrointestinal (upset stomach, diarrhea, abdominal pain).

ACEBUTOLOL; *Sectral, Monitan*	L3
Uses: Antihypertensive, beta blocker	B

AAP: Drugs associated with significant side effects and should be given with caution

T½= 3-4 hours;   **RID**= 3.6%;   **Oral** = 35-50%;   **MW**= 336

Clinical: Of the beta blockers, acebutolol produces rather significant levels in milk (10% of maternal dose). While thousands of breastfeeding mothers have taken this product safely, I would suggest the use of metoprolol instead, as its milk levels are quite low.

ACETAMINOPHEN; *Tempra, Tylenol, Paracetamol, Apo-Acetaminophen*	L1
Uses: Analgesic	B

AAP: Maternal medication usually compatible with breastfeeding

T½= 2 hours;   **RID**= 8.8% - 24.2%;   **Oral** = >85%;   **MW**= 151

Clinical: The use of acetaminophen in breastfeeding presents minimal risk to the infant and is probably safe. Patients should be advised to take no more than 4 grams/day due to the risk of liver toxicity.

ACETAZOLAMIDE; *Dazamide, Diamox, Acetazolam, Apo-Acetazolamide*	L2
Uses: Diuretic	C

AAP: Maternal medication usually compatible with breastfeeding

T½= 2.4-5.8 hours;   **RID**= 2.2%;   **Oral** = Complete;   **MW**= 222

Clinical: We have only limited data on this carbonic anhydrase inhibitor. Milk levels were low, only 1.3-2.1 mg/liter of milk. Infant plasma levels were 0.2 to 0.6 mg/L, or about 10-20 times less than the maternal levels. These levels are probably subclinical in infants.

ACETOHEXAMIDE; *Dymelor, Dimelor*	L3
Uses: Hypoglycemic agent	C
AAP: Not reviewed	

T½= 1.3-6 (metabolite) hours;   **RID**= ;   **Oral** = Good;   **MW**= 324

Clinical: We have little data on the sulfonylurea hypoglycemics in breastfed infants. If possible it is best to avoid them and use metformin or others that do not affect "normal" individuals blood glucose levels.

ACITRETIN; *Soriatane*	L5
Uses: Retinoid-like compound	X

AAP: Maternal medication usually compatible with breastfeeding

T½= 49 hours; **RID=** 1.8%; **Oral** = 72%; **MW=** 326

Clinical: This product is a long half-life retanoid. It is highly teratogenic and remains so for up to three years after exposure. Although it is not retained as long as etretinate, chronic use in breastfeeding mothers is not recommended.

ACYCLOVIR; *Zovirax, Lipsovir, Apo-Acyclovir, Aviraz*	L2
Uses: Antiviral	B

AAP: Maternal medication usually compatible with breastfeeding

T½= 2.4 hours; **RID=** 1.1% - 1.5%; **Oral** = 15-30%; **MW=** 225

Clinical: Acyclovir is used at high doses in infants all the time with only minor side effects. Its transfer into milk is relatively negligible. Mothers with lesions on the areola or nipple should not breastfeed. Other contiguous lesions should be thoroughly covered while breastfeeding.

ADALIMUMAB; *Humira*	L3
Uses: Anti-rheumatic, anti-tumor necrosis antibody	B

AAP: Not reviewed

T½= 2 weeks.; **RID=** ; **Oral** = Low; **MW=** 148,000

Clinical: IgG transfers into milk rather poorly. This IgG1 analog is even less likely to transfer. However, we do not have data on these products as of yet. It is rather unlikely these would affect a breastfeeding infant following oral ingestion at levels that are likely to be low.

ADAPALENE; *Differin*	L3
Uses: Topical acne remedy	C

AAP: Not reviewed

T½= ; RID= ; Oral = ; MW=

Clinical: This retinoid-like compound is virtually unabsorbed transcutaneously. Although milk levels have not been reported, they are likely to be undetectable due to low plasma levels in the mother.

ADEFOVIR DIPIVOXIL; *Hepsera*	L4

Uses: Anti-Hepatitis B Virus agent	C

AAP: Not reviewed

T½= 7.5 hours; RID= ; Oral = 59%; MW= 501

Clinical: Adofovir is a nucleotide analog which disrupts hepatitis B DNA replication. There are no data on its transfer into human milk, however milk levels will likely be low. Due to its chronic use, the risk of side effects in the breastfeeding infant is possibly significant. This product should not be used in breastfeeding mothers chronically until we know more. Adefovir is indicated for use in patients with lamivudine-resistant hepatitis B as well as na"ve patients.

ADENOSINE	L3

Uses: Adenosine Receptor Agonist	C

AAP: Not reviewed

T½= ; RID= ; Oral = ; MW= 267.2

Clinical: There are no adequate well controlled studies in breastfeeding. However, adenosine has a half-life <10 seconds and is not likely bioavailable long enough to enter the milk. Based on this information, it is probably safe to use in breastfeeding.

AIRBORNE	

Uses: HERBAL

AAP: Not reviewed

T½= ; RID= ; Oral = ; MW=

Clinical: Airborne contains Vits. A, C, E, K plus riboflavin, selenium, zinc sulfate, magenese, glutamine, lysine, mineral oil, sucralose, sorbitol, citric acid, NaHCO3, KHCO3, echinacea, schizonepeta ginger, chinese vitex, magnesium, zinc, Na, K, maltodextrin, Lonicera, Forsythia.

ALBENDAZOLE; *Albenza*	L3
Uses: Anthelminic for treatment of numerous varieties of worms	C
AAP: Not reviewed	
T½= 8 hours; **RID**= ; **Oral** = <5%; **MW**= 265	
Clinical: Albendazole is a commonly used anthelminic all over the world. It is poorly absorbed orally and milk levels would be undoubtedly low to nil. Normal doses for infants range from 400 mg daily to 10 mg/kg daily for 7 days. It would be extremely unlikely for levels present in milk to harm an infant.	

ALBUTEROL AND IPRATROPIUM BROMIDE; *DuoNeb*	L1
Uses: Bronchodilators	C
AAP: Not reviewed	
T½= ; **RID**= ; **Oral** = ; **MW**=	
Clinical: Both albuterol and ipratropium are relatively safe to use in breastfeeding. The inhaled dose has minimal systemic absorption and passage into human milk.	

ALBUTEROL; *Proventil, Novo-Salmol, Ventolin, Asmavent*	L1
Uses: Bronchodilator for asthma	C
AAP: Not reviewed	
T½= 3.8 hours; **RID**= ; **Oral** = 100%; **MW**= 239	
Clinical: Albuterol administered intranasally is safe in breastfeeding due to low systemic bioavailability (<10%). Oral administration of albuterol has a higher likelihood of transfering into milk, which may lead to tremors and excitement in the infant.	

ALCAFTADINE OPHTHALMIC SOLUTION; *Lastacaft*	L3
Uses: Topical H1 histamine receptor	B
AAP: Not reviewed	
T½= 2 hrs for the metabolite; **RID**= ; **Oral** = ; **MW**= 307.39	
Clinical: No breastfeeding studies available. Unlikely to be a problem for a breastfed infant due to minimal intraocular dose.	

ALEFACEPT; *Amevive*
L3

Uses: Immunosuppresant	**B**

AAP: Not reviewed

T½= 270 hours; **RID**= ; **Oral** = Nil; **MW**= 91,400

Clinical: This is a large molecular weight protein (91.4 kilodaltons) that is only administered by injection. It is indicated for moderate to severe plaque psoriasis. There are no data available on its transfer into human milk, but it is unlikely due to its large molecular weight. Further, it would be unabsorbed orally.

ALEMTUZUMAB; *Campath*
L3

Uses: Anti-leukemic agent	**C**

AAP: Not reviewed

T½= 12 days; **RID**= ; **Oral** = Nil; **MW**= 150,000

Clinical: After first week postpartum, alemtuzumab usage during breastfeeding poses minimal risk to the infant. It is highly unlikely that alemtuzumab transfers into milk since it is such a large molecule. No adverse effects are reported in breastfed infants.

ALENDRONATE SODIUM; *Fosamax*
L3

Uses: Inhibits bone resorption	**C**

AAP: Not reviewed

T½= <3 hours (plasma); **RID**= ; **Oral** = <0.7%; **MW**= 325

Clinical: At present, there are no data on the transfer of alendronate into human milk. Kinetics suggest that milk levels will be exceedingly low. However, although low, the risk of altering bone growth and remodeling in infants is possible if exposed to this product. Long-term exposure to this medication poses an unknown risk to a breastfeeding infant. Some caution is recommended.

ALFENTANIL; *Alfenta*
L2

Uses: Narcotic analgesic	**C**

AAP: Not reviewed

T½= 1-2 hours; **RID**= 0.4%; **Oral** = ; **MW**= 417

Clinical: Transfer of alfentanil in milk is minimal, and it is probably safe to use in breastfeeding. Observe for sedation, constipation, severe hypotension. Caution in infants with apnea, avoid usage.

ALISKIREN; *Tekturna, Valturna, Tekturna HCT*	L3
Uses: Renin inhibitor	C

AAP: Not reviewed

$T\frac{1}{2}$= 24 hours; **RID**= ; **Oral** = 3%; **MW**= 609

Clinical: This new renin inhibitor has not been studied in breastfeeding mothers. Milk levels are unreported, however its large molecular weight and low oral bioavailability will reduce the risk to a breastfeeding infant. Other antihypertensives that have some breastfeeding data are preferred at this time.

ALLERGY INJECTIONS	L1
Uses: Desensitizing injections	

AAP: Not reviewed

$T\frac{1}{2}$= ; **RID**= ; **Oral** = ; **MW**=

Clinical: Allergy injections are safe to use in breastfeeding. Transfer to milk is likely minimal. Observe for allergic reactions, although adverse effects are unlikely in the breastfed infant.

ALLOPURINOL; *Zyloprim, Lopurin, Alloprin, Apo-Allopurinol, Novo-Purol*	L2
Uses: Reduces uric acid levels	C

AAP: Maternal medication usually compatible with breastfeeding

$T\frac{1}{2}$= 1-3 hours (allopurinol); **RID**= 4.9%; **Oral** = 90%; **MW**= 136

Clinical: Levels in milk are low, and levels of the metabolite are higher in milk. Allopurinol usage during breastfeeding is probably safe. One infant that breastfed through 6 weeks of allopurinol therapy had no adverse effects. Observe for itching, fever, chills, N/V/D in the breastfed infant.

ALMOTRIPTAN; *Axert*	L3
Uses: Acute migraine treatment	C

AAP: Not reviewed

$T\frac{1}{2}$= 3-4 hours; **RID**= ; **Oral** = 80%; **MW**=

Clinical: We do not have data on transfer of almotriptan into human milk, although transfer into milk is likely from a pharmacokinetic standpoint. Observe for sedation, dry mouth in the breastfed infant. A suitable alternative is sumatriptan, of which we have more data on.

ALOE VERA; *Aloe Vera, Cape, Zanzibar, Socotrine*	L3
Uses: Extract from A. Vera	
AAP: Not reviewed	

$T\frac{1}{2}=$; **RID=** ; **Oral =** ; **MW=**

Clinical: Aloe vera is probably okay to use during breastfeeding if used acutely and topically. Caution is advised when used orally. No adverse effects have been reported in breastfed infants. Avoid oral use in breastfeeding mothers.

ALOSETRON; *Lotronex*	L3
Uses: Treatment of Irritable Bowel Syndrome	B
AAP: Not reviewed	

$T\frac{1}{2}=$ 1.5 hours; **RID=** ; **Oral =** 50-60%; **MW=**

Clinical: Alosetron is not well-studied in breastfeeding. It has low plasma levels and so the milk levels are likely low. Caution is advised since we know little about this product. Observe for constipation in the breastfed infant. Loperamide is a suitable alternative.

ALPHA- GALACTOSIDASE ENZYME; *Beano, Saint Ignatius-beans*	L3
Uses: Antiflatulant	
AAP: Not reviewed	

$T\frac{1}{2}=$; **RID=** ; **Oral =** ; **MW=** 101,000

Clinical: We have no data on alpha-galactosidase usage during breastfeeding. Since it is an enzyme naturally found in the body, it is probably okay when used sparingly. Effects are probably localized in the GI tract.

ALPRAZOLAM; *Xanax, Apo-Alpraz, Novo-Alprazol*	L3
Uses: Benzodiazepine antianxiety agent	D

AAP: Drugs whose effect on nursing infants is unknown but may be of concern

T½= 12-15 hours; **RID**= 8.5%; **Oral** = Complete; **MW**= 309

Clinical: Alprazolam is one of the preferred benzodiazepines for use in breastfeeding due to its relatively short half-life of 15 hours. A suitable alternative is lorazepam, which has a shorter half-life and is less addicting. Alprazolam is probably safe to use during breastfeeding when used short-term, intermittently, and low dose after the first week of life. Observe for sedation, poor feeding, irritability, crying, withdrawal symptoms in the breastfed infant.

ALTEPLASE; *Activase*	L3
Uses: Thrombolytic agent	C

AAP: Not reviewed

T½= 26-46 minutes; **RID**= ; **Oral** = Nil; **MW**= Large

Clinical: Alteplase is a large molecule that is unlikely to transfer into milk. Also, it is not orally absorbed, thus infants should be unaffected. Potential adverse effect is bleeding or bruising, however no adverse effects have been reported in the breastfed infant.

ALVIMOPAN; *Entereg*	L3
Uses: Peripheral opiate receptor blocker for postoperative ileus.	B

AAP: Not reviewed

T½= 10-17 hours; **RID**= ; **Oral** = 6%; **MW**= 460

Clinical: Alvimopan has low oral absorption and low plasma levels. Thus, levels in milk are probably minimal. One time usage or intermittent is probably okay in breastfeeding. Observe for constipation in the breastfed infant.

AMANTADINE; *Symmetrel, Symadine, Endantanine, Gen-Amantadine*	L3
Uses: Anti-viral and antiparkinsonian	C

AAP: Not reviewed

T½= 1-28 hours; **RID**= ; **Oral** = 86-94%; **MW**= 151

Clinical: Amantadine is a unique compound that has both antiviral activity against influenza A and is effective in treating Parkinsonian symptoms. Only trace amounts are believed to be secreted in milk although no reports are found. However, amantadine is known to suppress prolactin production and should not be used in breastfeeding mothers or at least should be used with caution while observing for milk suppression.

AMIKACIN; *Amikin*	L2
Uses: Aminoglycoside antibiotic	D

AAP: Not reviewed

T½= 2.3 hours; **RID**= ; **Oral** = Poor; **MW**= 586

Clinical: Only very small amounts are secreted into breastmilk. Following 100 and 200 mg IM doses, only trace amounts have been found in breastmilk and then in only 2 of 4 patients studied. In another study of 2-3 patients who received 100 mg IM, none to trace amounts were found in milk.

AMINOSALICYLIC ACID (PARA); *Paser, PAS, Tubasal, Nemasol*	L3
Uses: Antitubercular	C

AAP: Drugs associated with significant side effects and should be given with caution

T½= 1 hour; **RID**= 0.3%; **Oral** = >90%; **MW**= 153

Clinical: The concentrations of 5-ASA and its metabolite Acetyl-5-ASA present in milk appear too low to produce overt toxicity in most infants. Only one report of slight diarrhea in one infant has been reported.

AMIODARONE; *Cordarone*	L5
Uses: Strong antiarrhythmic agent	D

AAP: Drugs whose effect on nursing infants is unknown but may be of concern

T½= 26-107 days; **RID**= 43.1%; **Oral** = 22-86%; **MW**= 643

Clinical: The use of amiodarone in a breastfeeding mother is risky. This product would enter milk in significant quantities. It would subsequently be absorbed by infants and stored in their adipose tissue for long periods. If the mom discontinues amiodarone, prior to breastfeeding or shortely thereafter, or uses it only briefly (a few days), then the risk to the infant is probably minimal. But sustained and continued use during breastfeeding poses a high risk to an infant.

AMITRIPTYLINE; *Elavil, Endep, Limbitrol, Apo-Amitriptyline, Novo-Tryptin*	L2
Uses: Tricyclic antidepressant	C

AAP: Drugs whose effect on nursing infants is unknown but may be of concern

T½= 31-46 hours; **RID=** 1.9% - 2.8%; **Oral =** Complete; **MW=** 277

Clinical: No untoward effects have been noted in numerous studies and infants. Side effects in adult patients are significant including many anticholinergic problems, such as constipation, dry mouth, blurred vision. Patient compliance is poor due to these problems. Quite toxic in overdose, so advise patients to keep away from children.

AMLODIPINE BESYLATE; *Norvasc*	L3
Uses: Antihypertensive, calcium channel blocker	C

AAP: Not reviewed

T½= 30-50 hours; **RID=** ; **Oral =** 64-65%; **MW=** 408

Clinical: No data are currently available on transfer of amlodipine into breastmilk. Because most calcium channel blockers (CCB) readily transfer into milk, we should assume the same for this drug. Use caution if administering to lactating women.

AMOXAPINE; *Asendin*	L2
Uses: Tricyclic antidepressant	C

AAP: Drugs whose effect on nursing infants is unknown but may be of concern

T½= 8 hours (parent); **RID=** 0.6%; **Oral =** 18-54%; **MW=** 314

Clinical: Amoxapine is probably safe to use during breastfeeding. Transfer to breast milk seems to be minimal, and there are no reports of adverse effects in breastfed infants. Observe for sedation. SSRIs as a class like sertraline are preferred for treatment of depression during breastfeeding.

AMOXICILLIN + CLAVULANATE; *Augmentin, Clavulin*	L1
Uses: Penicillin antibiotic, extended spectrum	B
AAP: Not reviewed	
T½= 1.7 hours; **RID**= 0.9%; **Oral** = 89%; **MW**= 365	
Clinical: Observe for minor side effects including rash, irritability, constipation, or diarrhea.	

AMOXICILLIN; *Larotid, Amoxil, Apo-Amoxi, Novamoxin*	L1
Uses: Penicillin antibiotic	B
AAP: Maternal medication usually compatible with breastfeeding	
T½= 1.7 hours; **RID**= 1%; **Oral** = 89%; **MW**= 365	
Clinical: Amoxicillin is commonly used in neonates and infants and is safe to use during breastfeeding. No adverse effects have been reported in breastfed infants.	

AMPHOTERICIN B; *Fungizone, Amphotec, Ambisome, Resteclin*	L3
Uses: Antifungal	B
AAP: Not reviewed	
T½= 15 days; **RID**= ; **Oral** = <9%; **MW**= 924	
Clinical: Levels in milk are probably low, although unpublished. Further, virtually none would be absorbed orally in an infant.	

AMPICILLIN + SULBACTAM; *Unasyn*	L1
Uses: Penicillin antibiotic with extended spectrum.	B
AAP: Not reviewed	
T½= 1.3 hours; **RID**= 0.5% - 1.5%; **Oral** = 60%; **MW**= 349	
Clinical: Small amount may be present in milk. Only likely problem is change in gut flora. Observe for candida overgrowth or diarrhea.	

AMPICILLIN; *Polycillin, Omnipen, Apo-Ampi, Novo-Ampicillin, NuAmpi, Penbriton*	L1
Uses: Penicillin antibiotic	B
AAP: Not reviewed	
T½= 1.3 hours; **RID=** 0.17-0.51%; **Oral =** 50%; **MW=** 349	
Clinical: Ampicillin usage during breastfeeding is safe. The levels in milk are minimal, and there have been no reports of adverse effects in breastfed infants. Observe for diarrhea, hypersensitivity to penicillin, rash.	

ANAGRELIDE HYDROCHLORIDE; *Agrylin*	L4
Uses: Platelet-reducing agent	C
AAP: Not reviewed	
T½= 1.3 hours; **RID=** ; **Oral =** 70%; **MW=** 310	
Clinical: This product is orally absorbed, rather smaller in molecular weight, and some will probably enter the milk compartment. Prolonged exposure in infants could be problematic and I would not recommend breastfeeding with the chronic use of this product.	

ANAKINRA; *Kineret*	L3
Uses: Anti-rheumatic	B
AAP: Not reviewed	
T½= 4-6 hours; **RID=** ; **Oral =** Nil; **MW=** 17,300	
Clinical: Anakinra is a large molecular weight protein. It is unlikely to enter milk in clinically relevant amounts, or to be orally bioavailable in the infant. But some proteins are known to enter milk from the plasma compartment. Infants should be observed for risk of GI infections.	

ANIDULAFUNGIN; *Eraxis*	L3
Uses: Antifungal	C
AAP: Not reviewed	
T½= 27 hours; **RID=** ; **Oral =** Nil; **MW=** 1140.3	
Clinical: This product is not likely to enter milk. It is >99% protein bound, has a huge volume of distribution, and massive molecular weight. It would not be orally bioavailable.	

ANTHRALIN; *Anthra-Derm, Drithocreme, Dritho-Scalp, Micanol, Anthraforte, Anthranol, Anthrascalp*	L3
Uses: Anti-psoriatic	C
AAP: Not reviewed	
T½= Brief; **RID=** ; **Oral** = Complete; **MW=** 226	

Clinical: Anthralin when applied topically is absorbed into the surface layers of the skin and only minimal amounts enter the systemic circulation. That absorbed is rapidly excreted via the kidneys almost instantly; plasma levels are very low to undetectable. No data are available on its transfer into human milk. When placed directly on lesions on the areola or nipple, breastfeeding should be discouraged. Another similar anthraquinone is Senna (laxative), which even in high doses does not enter milk. While undergoing initial intense treatment, it would perhaps be advisable to interrupt breastfeeding temporarily, but this may be overly conservative. Observe the infant for diarrhea

ANTHRAX (BACILLUS ANTHRACIS); *Anthrax Infection, Bacillus Anthracis*	L5
Uses: Anthrax infection	
AAP: Not reviewed	
T½= ; **RID=** ; **Oral** = ; **MW=**	

Clinical: Follow CDC guidelines for treatment.

ANTHRAX VACCINE; *Anthrax Vaccine*	L3
Uses: Vaccination	C
AAP: Not reviewed	
T½= ; **RID=** ; **Oral** = ; **MW=**	

Clinical: There are no data or indications relative to its use in breastfeeding mothers. While it consists primarily of protein fragments of anthrax bacteria, it is very unlikely any would transfer into milk or even be bioavailable in the infant. The CDC states that, "No data suggest increased risk for side effects or temporally related adverse events associated with receipt of anthrax vaccine by breast-feeding women or breast-fed children. Administration of nonliving vaccines (e.g., anthrax vaccine) during breast-feeding is not medically contraindicated."

ANTIHEMOPHILIC FACTOR-VON WILLEBRAND FACTOR COMPLEX; *Alphanate, Humate-P, Wilate*	L3

Uses: Antihemophilic agent	C

AAP: Not reviewed

T½= 10-12 hours; **RID=** ; **Oral =** Nil; **MW=** 264,726

Clinical: This is a large molecular weight protein that is unlikely to enter milk or be orally bioavailable. It should pose no risk to a breastfed infant.

ANTIPYRINE; *Antipyrine*	L4

Uses: Analgesic, antipyretic	C

AAP: Not reviewed

T½= ; **RID=** 8.3% - 25%; **Oral =** ; **MW=** 188

Clinical: This product is no longer used in the USA due to high incidence of fatal bone marrow toxicity. In a group of 7 breastfeeding mothers who were receiving a single oral dose of 18 mg/kg of antipyrine in solution, peak levels in milk ranged from 10-30 mg/L. The average amount of antipyrine available to the nursing infant was estimated at 6.4 mg/24 hours (range 3.0-11.1 mg).

ARFORMOTEROL TARTRATE; *Brovana*	L3

Uses: Beta-2 agonist	C

AAP: Not reviewed

T½= 26 hours; **RID=** ; **Oral =** ; **MW=** 494.5

Clinical: This long-acting beta agonist is similar to the other selective beta-2 agonists, although it is indicated for COPD. Minimal plasma levels suggest levels in milk will be minimal as well.

ARGATROBAN; *Argatroban*	L4

Uses: Synthetic direct thrombin inhibitor: anticoagulant	B

AAP: Not reviewed

T½= 39-51 minutes; **RID=** ; **Oral =** Unknown; **MW=** 526

Clinical: It is not known if this product is orally bioavailable, but probably not. The presence of this product in milk could potentially induce GI hemorrhage in weak or susceptible infants including newborns, premature infants, infants with NEC, and other infants. Extreme caution is recommended until we know levels present in milk and more about its GI stability, absorption. It has a low volume of distribution. No data are available on its transfer to human milk

ARGININE; *L-Arginine, Arginine*	L3
Uses: Amino Acid; test for Growth Hormone release	B

AAP: Not reviewed

T½= <2 hours; **RID=** ; **Oral** = 70%; **MW=** 174

Clinical: No reports of its transfer into human milk are available. Most importantly, we do not know if high doses of oral L-Arginine (> 30gm/day) subsequently increase Arginine levels in milk, although it would seem likely. As this product has limited usefulness in most patients, its use at high doses in breastfeeding mothers should be avoided until milk levels are reported. Doses as high as 30 gm/day have been generally well tolerated in adults with the most common adverse effects of nausea and diarrhea being reported.

ARIPIPRAZOLE; *Abilify, Abilitat*	L3
Uses: Antipsychotic	C

AAP: Not reviewed

T½= 75 hours; **RID=** 1%; **Oral** = 87%; **MW=** 448

Clinical: Only one small case report has been found. Milk and plasma levels were unfortunately taken almost at trough. Milk/plasma ratio is reported to be 0.2 and milk levels were 13 and 14 ug/Liter of milk. Using this data, the RID is about 1%. Its probably higher as the peak with this drug occurs at 3-5 hours, but due to its long half-life, the peak is probably not that high at steady state. I've received several cases of somnolent babies in mothers using this product. Some caution is recommended until we know more.

ARMODAFINIL; *Nuvigil*	L4
Uses: Wakefulness-Promoting Agent	C

AAP: Not reviewed

T½= 15 hours; **RID=** ; **Oral** = ; **MW=** 273

Clinical: We have no data on the transfer of armodafinil into breast milk, however the low molecular weight and its ability to transfer to the CNS, suggest it is likely. Methylphenidate is a suitable alternative for treatment of narcolepsy in breastfeeding.

ASCORBIC ACID; *Ascorbicap, Cecon, Cevi-Bid, Ce-Vi-Sol, Vitamin C*	L1
Uses: Vitamin C	A
AAP: Not reviewed	
T½= ; **RID=** ; **Oral** = Complete; **MW=** 176	

Clinical: Ascorbic acid transfer into milk is controlled in large part by the controlled levels in the plasma compartment. Even following high doses, ascorbic acid levels don't rise too much in milk. Recommend normal RDA in mothers. Do not use excessive levels while breastfeeding.

ASPARTAME; *Nutrasweet, Equal, Sugar Twin*	L1
Uses: Artificial sweetener	B
AAP: Not reviewed	
T½= ; **RID=** ; **Oral** = Complete; **MW=** 294	

Clinical: Milk levels are too low to produce significant side effects in normal infants. Contraindicated in infants with proven phenylketonuria. Maternal ingestion of 50 mg/kg aspartame will approximately double (2.3 to 4.8 µmol/dL) aspartate milk levels. Phenylalanine milk levels similarly increased from 0.5 to 2.3 µmol/dL.

ASPIRIN; *Anacin, Aspergum, Empirin, Genprin, Arthritis Foundation Pain Reliever, Ecotrin, Bayer, Alka-Seltzer, Bufferin, Coryphen, Ecotrin, Novasen, Entrophen*	L3
Uses: Salicylate analgesic	C
AAP: Drugs associated with significant side effects and should be given with caution	
T½= 2.5-7 hours; **RID=** 2.5% - 10.8%; **Oral** = 80-100%; **MW=** 180	

Clinical: Aspirin is rapidly metabolized to salicylic acid. However, the acetylated form of aspirin does rapidly chelate with platelets prior to its metabolism. Aspirin is certainly implicated in Reye syndrome, but most often in older children (not infants) who have a viral illness such as flu or chickenpox. Even when present at small plasma levels in these children, it was implicated in Reye syndrome. However, the amount in breastmilk is incredibly low even following large therapeutic doses. The amount in milk following low (82 mg) doses is probably infinitesimally low. In these cases the risk to the infant is probably remote. The urgent need for low-dose aspirin in a breastfeeding mother would require a major discussion of the risk vs benefit.

ATENOLOL; *Tenoretic, Tenormin, Apo-Atenolol*	L3
Uses: Beta adrenergic blocker, antihyertensive	D

AAP: Drugs associated with significant side effects and should be given with caution

T½= 6.1 hours; **RID=** 6.6%; **Oral =** 50-60%; **MW=** 266

Clinical: Atenolol is one of the few beta blockers that produces significant adverse effects in breastfed infants. Observe for bradycardia, weakness, hypotension, cyanosis, tiredness in the breastfed infant. More suitable beta blockers are metoprolol and propranolol.

ATOMOXETINE; *Strattera*	L4
Uses: Stimulant for treatment of ADHD	C

AAP: Not reviewed

T½= 5.2 hours; **RID=** ; **Oral =** 63-94%; **MW=** 291

Clinical: No data are available on the transfer of Atomoxetine into human milk. Because this is a lipophilic, neuroactive drug, there is some potential risk coincident with its use in a breastfeeding mother, and mothers should probably be cautioned about its use while breastfeeding.

ATOVAQUONE AND PROGUANIL; *Malarone*	L3
Uses: Antimalarials	C

AAP: Not reviewed

T½= ; **RID=** ; **Oral =** ; **MW=**

Clinical: Only trace quantities of proguanil were found in human milk. Further, while the pharmacokinetics of proguanil is similar in adults and pediatric patients, the elimination half-life of atovaquone is much shorter in pediatric patients (1-2 days) than in adult patients (2-3 days). Elimination half-life ranges from 32 to 84 hours for atovaquone and 12 to 21 hours for proguanil; the half-life of cycloguanil is approximately 14 hours.

ATROPINE; *Belladonna, Atropine, Atropine Minims, Atropisol, Isopto-Atropine*	L3
Uses: Anticholinergic, drying agent	C

AAP: Maternal medication usually compatible with breastfeeding

T½= 4.3 hours; RID= ; Oral = 90%; MW= 289

Clinical: Only small amounts are believed secreted in milk. Effects may be highly variable. Slight absorption together with enhanced neonatal sensitivity creates hazardous potential. Use caution. Avoid if possible but not definitely contraindicated.

AZAPROPAZONE	L2
Uses: Analgesic	C

AAP: Maternal medication usually compatible with breastfeeding

T½= 13-14 hours; RID= 2.1%; Oral = 83%; MW=

Clinical: In a study of 4 patients each received 600 mg IV within 2 hours after giving birth and thereafter, they received 600 mg twice daily. Milk levels of azapropazone were measured on days 4 and 6 postpartum. The amount of azapropazone excreted in the breast milk within 12 h ranged from 0.2 mg to 1.3 mg (mean 0.8 mg in 12 h) or an average milk concentration of 2.43 µg/mL. The volume of milk produced during this 12 hour period averaged 329 mL. The relative infant dose over 24 hours would be 2.1% of the maternal dose. The authors did not report side effects in the infants.

AZATHIOPRINE; *Imuran*	L3
Uses: Immunosuppressive agent	D

AAP: Not reviewed

T½= 0.6 hour; RID= 0.07% - 0.3%; Oral = 41-44%; MW= 277

Clinical: The transport of 6-mercaptopurine into human milk is apparently quite low. However, this is a strong immunosuppressant and some caution is still recommended if it is used in a breastfeeding mother. Monitor the infant closely for signs of immunosuppression, leukopenia, thrombocytopenia, hepatotoxicity, pancreatitis, and other symptoms of 6-mercaptopurine exposure. The risks to the infant are probably low.

AZELAIC ACID; *Azelex, Finevin*	**L3**
Uses: Topical treatment of acne	B

AAP: Not reviewed

T½= 45 minutes; **RID**= ; **Oral** = ; **MW**= 188

Clinical: Small amounts of azelaic acid are normally present in human milk. Azelaic acid is only modestly absorbed via skin (<4%), and it is rapidly metabolized. The amount absorbed does not change the levels normally found in plasma nor milk. Due to its poor penetration into plasma and rapid half-life (45 min), it is not likely to penetrate milk or produce untoward effects in a breastfed infant.

AZELASTINE; *Astelin, Optivar, Astepro*	**L3**
Uses: Antihistamine	C

AAP: Not reviewed

T½= 22 hours; **RID**= ; **Oral** = 80%; **MW**= 418

Clinical: Azelastine is an antihistamine for oral, intranasal and ophthalmic administration. Ophthalmically, it is effective for allergic conjunctivitis (itchy eyes). No data are available on the transfer of azelastine into human milk. The doses used intranasally and ophthalmically are so low that it is extremely unlikely to produce clinically relevant levels in human milk. However, this is an extremely bitter product. It is possible that even miniscule amounts in milk could alter the taste of milk leading to rejection by the infant.

AZITHROMYCIN; *Zithromax*	**L2**
Uses: Antibiotic, macrolide	B

AAP: Not reviewed

T½= 48-68 hours; **RID**= 5.9%; **Oral** = 37%; **MW**= 749

Clinical: The predicted dose of azithromycin received by the infant would be approximately 0.4 mg/kg/day. This would suggest that the level of azithromycin ingested by a breastfeeding infant is not clinically relevant.

AZTREONAM; *Azactam*	L2

Uses: Antibiotic   B

AAP: Maternal medication usually compatible with breastfeeding

$T\frac{1}{2}$= 1.7 hours; **RID**= 0.2% - 1%; **Oral** = <1%; **MW**= 435

Clinical: The manufacturer reports that less than 1% of a maternal dose is transferred into milk. Due to poor oral absorption (<1%), no untoward effects would be expected in nursing infants, aside from changes in GI flora. An infant would ingest approximately <0.03% of the maternal dose per day (not weight adjusted).

BACITRACIN	L3

Uses: OTC Antibiotic

AAP: Not reviewed

$T\frac{1}{2}$= ; **RID**= ; **Oral** = ; **MW**=

Clinical: There are no adequate and well- controlled studies or case reports in breast feeding women. However this product is not overly hazardous and is unlikely to harm an infant.

BACLOFEN; *Lioresal, Atrofen, Novo-Baclofen, Apo-Baclofen*	L2

Uses: Skeletal muscle relaxant   C

AAP: Maternal medication usually compatible with breastfeeding

$T\frac{1}{2}$= 3-4 hours; **RID**= 6.9%; **Oral** = Complete; **MW**= 214

Clinical: Baclofen inhibits spinal reflexes and is used to reverse spasticity associated with multiple sclerosis or spinal cord lesions. Animal studies indicate baclofen inhibits prolactin release and may inhibit lactation. It is quite unlikely that baclofen administered intrathecally would be secreted into milk in significant quantities.

BALSALAZIDE DISODIUM; *Colazal*	L3

Uses: Antiinflammatory drug for ulcerative colitis   B

AAP: Not reviewed

T½= ; **RID=** ; **Oral** = <1%; **MW**= 437

Clinical: This is a prodrug of mesalamine. Although it is more expensive, it may be useful in patients unable to tolerate olsalazine or mesalamine. Mesalamine transfer to milk is documented to be about 7-8%. At least one case of watery diarrhea has been reported with mesalamine. Some caution is recommended, but this agent can probably be used with supervision in breastfeeding mothers.

BECLOMETHASONE; *Vanceril, Beclovent, Beconase, Becotide, Qvar, Propaderm, Becloforte*	**L2**
Uses: Intranasal, intrapulmonary steroid	C

AAP: Not reviewed

T½= 15 hours; **RID=** ; **Oral** = 90% (oral); **MW**= 409

Clinical: Beclomethasone is a potent steroid that is generally used via inhalation in asthma or via intranasal administration for allergic rhinitis. Intranasal absorption is generally minimal. Due to small doses administered, absorption into maternal plasma is extremely small. Therefore, it is unlikely that these doses would produce clinical significance in a breastfeeding infant.

BENAZEPRIL HCL; *Lotensin, Lotrel*	**L2**
Uses: Antihypertensive, ACE inhibitor	D

AAP: Not reviewed

T½= 10-11 hours; **RID=** ; **Oral** = 37%; **MW**= 424

Clinical: An ACE inhibitor, benazepril levels in milk are extremely low. In one study milk levels are in the nanogram/liter range (Cmax= 0.92 ng/L), hardly measurable. My estimates suggest the RID is 0.00005% of the weight-adjusted maternal dose.

BENDROFLUMETHIAZIDE; *Naturetin*	**L4**
Uses: Thiazide diuretic	C

AAP: Maternal medication usually compatible with breastfeeding

T½= 3-3.9 hours; **RID=** ; **Oral** = Complete; **MW**= 421

Clinical: Not generally recommended in breastfeeding mothers. Can suppress lactation.

BENZALKONIUM CHLORIDE	L3
Uses: OTC antimicrobial, skin protectant	
AAP: Not reviewed	
T½= ; **RID=** ; **Oral =** ; **MW=** variable	
Clinical: There are no adequate and well-controlled studies in lactating women. Not absorbed systemically.	

BENZOCAINE; *Orajel, Auralgan*	L3
Uses: Local Anesthetic	C
AAP: Not reviewed	
T½= ; **RID=** ; **Oral =** ; **MW=**	
Clinical: There are no adequate and well-controlled studies or case reports in breast feeding women. Probably safe used topically or orally.	

BENZONATATE; *Tessalon Perles*	L3
Uses: Antitussive	C
AAP: Advise not to breastfeed	
T½= <8 hours; **RID=** ; **Oral =** Good; **MW=** 603	
Clinical: Benzonatate is a non-narcotic cough suppressant similar to the local anesthetic tetracaine. It is of questionable efficacy. No data are available on its transfer to milk. However, in overdose (as little as 2 capsules in a child), this is a very dangerous product, leading to seizures with cardiac arrest and death, particularly in children.	

BENZOYL PEROXIDE	L3
Uses: Peroxide Antimicrobial	C
AAP: Not reviewed	
T½= ; **RID=** ; **Oral =** ; **MW=** 242.23	
Clinical: Because only about 5% of topically applied benzoyl peroxide is absorbed, it is thought to be of low risk to a nursing infant.	

BENZTROPINE MESYLATE; *Cogentin*	L3
Uses: Anticholinergic	C
AAP: Not reviewed	

T½= Long; **RID=** ; **Oral** = Poor; **MW=** 307

Clinical: Benztropine is a tertiary amine with poor oral absorption. It has a long (but unpublished) half-life as it effects last up to 24 hours. While we have no data on its transfer into human milk, due to its structure, it is probably minimal. Nevertheless, the potential for anticholinergic symptoms is significant and the prescribing clinician should observe the infant closely for symptoms.

BEPRIDIL HCL; *Vascor, Bepadin*	L4
Uses: Antihypertensive, calcium channel blocker	C
AAP: Not reviewed	

T½= 42 hours; **RID=** ; **Oral** = 60%; **MW=** 367

Clinical: This is a typical calcium channel blocker. We have little or no data on this product and other CCBs are much preferred with better data. See nifedipine, nimodipine, or verapamil.

BETAMETHASONE; *Betameth, Celestone, Beben, Betadermetnesol, Diprolene, Dipr*	L3
Uses: Synthetic corticosteroid	C
AAP: Not reviewed	

T½= 5.6 hours; **RID=** ; **Oral** = Complete; **MW=** 392

Clinical: In small doses, most steroids are certainly not contraindicated in nursing mothers. Whenever possible use low-dose alternatives such as aerosols or inhalers. Following administration, wait at least 4 hours if possible prior to feeding infant to reduce exposure. With high doses (>40 mg/day), particularly for long periods, steroids could potentially produce problems in infant growth and development, although we have absolutely no data in this area, or which doses would pose problems. Brief applications of high dose steroids are probably not contraindicated as the overall exposure is low. With prolonged high dose therapy, the infant should be closely monitored for growth and development.

BETAXOLOL; *Kerlone, Betoptic*	L3
Uses: Beta blocker antihypertensive	C
AAP: Not reviewed	

T½= 14-22 hours; **RID=** ; **Oral** = 89%; **MW=** 307

Clinical: There is little or no data on this beta blocker. The manufacturer states that no beta blockade is evident following its used ophthalmically. Thus it is probably safe to use in breastfeeding mothers.

BETHANECHOL CHLORIDE; *Urabeth, Urecholine, Duvoid, Urecholine*	L4
Uses: Cholinergic stimulant-agonist for urinary retention	C

AAP: Not reviewed

T½= 1-2 hours; **RID**= ; **Oral** = Poor; **MW**= 197

Clinical: The data on this drug in breastfeeding is somewhat obscure. This product is poorly absorbed orally, but breastfeeding infants could be exceedingly sensitive to the cholinergic-agonist effect of this product. It would be observed as diarrhea, gastric cramping and other typical cholinergic symptoms. Some caution is recommended with this product since we know so little about it in breastfeeding mothers.

BEVACIZUMAB; *Avastin*	L3
Uses: Immune modulator, VEGF inhibitor	C

AAP: Not reviewed

T½= 20 days; **RID**= ; **Oral** = Nil; **MW**= 149,000

Clinical: While we have no reports on its use in breastfeeding mothers, size alone would largely exclude it from the milk compartment. The intravitreal use of this drug is probably compatible with breastfeeding. The systemic use of this drug would not be compatible with breastfeeding.

BIMATOPROST; *Lumigan*	L3
Uses: Antiglaucoma agent	C

AAP: Not reviewed

T½= 45 minutes; **RID**= ; **Oral** = ; **MW**= 415

Clinical: Low plasma levels and higher protein binding suggest this product is unlikely to enter the milk compartment.

BISACODYL; *Bisacodyl, Dacodyl, Dulcolax, Fleet, Alophen, Correctol, Carter's Little Pills, Bisacolax, Dulcolax, Laxit, Apo-Bisacodyl*	**L2**
Uses: Laxative	**C**

AAP: Not reviewed

T½= 16 hours; **RID=** ; **Oral** = < 5%; **MW=** 361

Clinical: Bisacodyl effects are mainly localized in the GI tract, and GI absorption is poor. Thus, transfer to milk is highly unlikely. Bisacodyl is likely safe to use during breastfeeding. Avoid chronic usage. Observe for diarrhea, GI cramping in the breastfed infant, although risk is minimal.

BISMUTH SUBSALICYLATE; *Pepto-Bismol, Bismuth Liquid*	**L3**
Uses: Antisecretory, antimicrobial salt	**C**

AAP: Drugs whose effect on nursing infants is unknown but may be of concern

T½= ; **RID=** ; **Oral** = Poor; **MW=** 362

Clinical: Poor absorption limits effects of bismuth subsalicylate to the GI tract. Theoretical risk of Reye's syndrome in the breastfed infant, although there have been no reports of adverse effects. Limited use intermittently should be okay during breastfeeding.

BISOPROLOL; *Ziac, Zebeta*	**L3**
Uses: Beta-adrenergic antihypertensive	**C**

AAP: Not reviewed

T½= 9-12 hours; **RID=** ; **Oral** = 80%; **MW=** 325

Clinical: A typical beta blocker, bisoprolol transfer into milk is not published, but is believed to be low. Because atenolol and acebutolol have been associated with hypotension and apnea in infants, I suggest you use metoprolol instead since we know its levels in milk are very low. There are no adequate data to show that this beta blocker (bisoprolol) is any better than any other.

BLACK COHOSH; *Bane berry, Black Snakeroot, Bugbane, Squaw root, Rattle root*	**L4**
Uses: Herbal estrogenic compound	**X**

AAP: Not reviewed

T½= ; RID= ; Oral = ; MW=

Clinical: No data are available on the transfer of Black Cohosh into human milk, but due to its estrogenic activity, it could lower milk production although this is not known at this time. Caution is recommended in breastfeeding mothers. Use for more than 6 months is not recommended.

BLESSED THISTLE; *Blessed Thistle*	L3
Uses: Anorexic, antidiarrheal, febrifuge	

AAP: Not reviewed

T½= ; RID= ; Oral = ; MW=

Clinical: While this product has been suggested to be a galactagogue, no clinical data really support this use. The German E commission, nor many other herbal textbooks list it as a galactagogue. However, it is relatively nontoxic and it is unlikely to harm a breastfeeding infant, although this is rather poor justification for using it in a breastfeeding mother.

BLUE COHOSH; *Blue ginseng, Squaw root, Papoose root, Yellow ginseng*	L5
Uses: Uterine stimulant	X

AAP: Not reviewed

T½= ; RID= ; Oral = ; MW=

Clinical: Blue cohosh is a strong myocardial toxin and should never be used in breastfeeding mothers, or pregnant mothers.

BORAGE; *Borage, Borage oil, Beebread, Bee plant, Burrage, Starflower, Ox*	L5
Uses: Herbal expectorant, tonic, galactogogue	X

AAP: Not reviewed

T½= ; RID= ; Oral = ; MW=

Clinical: Borage oil or other products may contain powerful and dangerous pyrrolizidine alkaloids. Comfrey tea and other herbals may contain hepatotoxic alkaloids (like Borage), or myocardial toxins such as with Blue Cohosh. Borage is known to contain amabiline which is a known hepatotoxin. Although amabiline-free products are available, great caution is recommended. The potential hazards of this product do not warrant its use in breastfeeding mothers.

BOSENTAN; *Tracleer*	L4
Uses: Endothelin antagonist	X

AAP: Not reviewed

T½= 5 hours; **RID**= ; **Oral** = 50%; **MW**= 569

Clinical: This is a hazardous product. Although milk levels are likely low, chronic administration of even low levels could be hazardous. Liver toxicity occurs in 11% of patients. I would not recommend breastfeeding with this product until we have published milk levels.

BOTULINUM TOXIN; *Botox, Xeomin*	L3
Uses: Botulism poisoning and cosmetic procedures	C

AAP: Not reviewed

T½= ; **RID**= ; **Oral** = ; **MW**=

Clinical: When used in the form of Botox, and injected properly, it is extremely unlikely to ever enter the plasma or milk compartment. A brief interruption of a few hours to ascertain that none has entered the plasma would all but eliminate any possible complications in a breastfeeding mother. Further, because this product is so large, it would have an extremely difficult time entering the milk compartment, which is shown by the lack of entry reference one.

BRIMONIDINE; *Alphagan*	L3
Uses: Use to treat ocular hypertension	B

AAP: Not reviewed

T½= 3 hours; **RID**= ; **Oral** = ; **MW**= 442

Clinical: No data are available on the transfer of this alpha blocker into human milk. Plasma levels are even unreported, but we know some is retained in the plasma compartment from the reported side effect profiles. If used in breastfeeding mothers, the infant should be closely monitored for alpha blockade.

BROMOCRIPTINE MESYLATE; *Parlodel, Apo-Bromocriptine*	L5
Uses: Inhibits prolactin secretion	B

AAP: Drugs associated with significant side effects and should be given with caution

T½= 50 hours; **RID**= ; **Oral** = <28%; **MW**= 654

Clinical: In general this product profoundly reduces prolactin levels. Although it is a risky product to use due to numerous side effects, it can still be used to suppress excessively high prolactin levels in breastfeeding mothers. Levels can be titrated down to a suitable level and still allow lactation to ensue, although cabergoline is still safer and recommended for this purpose.

BROMPHENIRAMINE; *Dimetane, Brombay, Dimetapp, Bromfed*	**L3**
Uses: Antihistamine	**C**
AAP: Not reviewed	

T½= 24.9 hours; **RID**= ; **Oral** = Complete; **MW**= 319

Clinical: Brompheniramine has not been adequately studied in breastfeeding mothers, although some reports exist suggesting it might produce problems in some infants. Caution is recommended with this product, although the side effects are probably remote and minimal.

BUDESONIDE INHALED; *Rhinocort, Pulmicort Respules, Symbicort*	**L1**
Uses: Corticosteroid	**C**
AAP: Not reviewed	

T½= 2.8 hours; **RID**= 0.3%; **Oral** = 10.7% (oral); **MW**= 430

Clinical: Budesonide, however used, is a preferred steroid for breastfeeding women. It is rapidly cleared by the liver. It is poorly absorbed orally. And it produces the least HPA axis suppression when compared with many of the other oral steroids (predisone(20mg/d)=78% vs budesonide(9mg/d)=45% suppression of HPA). Steroids in general due to structural problems, enter milk poorly. Maternal use via intranasal or inhalation are no problem for a breastfeeding infant.

BUDESONIDE ORAL; *Entocort EC*	**L3**
Uses: Corticosteroid	**C**
AAP: Not reviewed	

T½= 2-3.6 hours; **RID**= ; **Oral** = 9-21%; **MW**= 430

Clinical: Budesonide orally administered should present minimal risk to the breastfed infant. The effect of budesonide oral is mainly local in the GI tract, minimal levels are detected in plasma. Thus, transfer to milk is probably minimal. There have been no reports of adverse effects in breastfed infants. Observe for impaired bone growth.

BUMETANIDE; *Bumex, Burinex*	L3
Uses: Loop diuretic	C
AAP: Not reviewed	
T½= 1-1.5; **RID**= ; **Oral** = ; **MW**= 364	
Clinical: Bumetanide is a potent loop diuretic and a poor alternative to furosemide. Use furosemide if needed as its transfer into milk is low, and its oral bioavailability in infants is quite low.	

BUPIVACAINE; *Marcaine*	L2
Uses: Epidural, local anesthetic	C
AAP: Not reviewed	
T½= 2.7 hours; **RID**= 0.9%; **Oral** = ; **MW**= 288	
Clinical: Bupivacaine transfer into milk is negligible. When it is used early postpartum, the minimal amount of milk secreted (30cc/day) and the limited amount present in milk, would all but preclude any toxicity in an infant. The infant is exposed to more in utero than via milk.	

BUPRENORPHINE + NALOXONE; *Suboxone*	L3
Uses: Opiate withdrawal	C
AAP: Not reviewed	
T½= ; **RID**= ; **Oral** = ; **MW**=	
Clinical: Naloxone is poorly absorbed orally and buprenorphine is only 31% absorbed. It is unlikely breast milk levels will be significant. See individual monographs on these two drugs.	

BUPRENORPHINE; *Buprenex, Subutex*	L2
Uses: Narcotic analgesic	C
AAP: Not reviewed	
T½= 23-30 h sublingual; **RID**= 1.9%; **Oral** = 31%; **MW**= 504	

Clinical: Studies thus far clearly show buprenorphine levels in milk are subclinical. Less than 2% of the dose transfers into milk and less than a third of this would be absorbed orally.

BUPROPION; *Wellbutrin, Zyban, Aplenzin, Wellbutrin*	L3
Uses: Antidepressant, smoking deterrent	C

AAP: Drugs whose effect on nursing infants is unknown but may be of concern

T½= 8-24 hours; **RID=** 0.2% - 2%; **Oral** = 85%; **MW=** 240

Clinical: Of the infants studied thus far, no bupropion has been detected in the infant's plasma compartment. However, one case of possible seizure has been reported. The author has had at least 3 case reports in which bupropion may have suppressed the mothers milk supply. Observe closely for changes in the mothers milk production.

BUSPIRONE; *BuSpar, Apo-Buspirone, Novo-Buspirone*	L3
Uses: Antianxiety medication	B

AAP: Not reviewed

T½= 2-3 hours; **RID=** ; **Oral** = 90%; **MW=** 386

Clinical: We have no data on buspirone transfer into milk. However, it appears to be a suitable alternative to benzodiazepines as an antianxiolytic since it has a short half-life and is less sedating.

BUSULFAN; *Myleran*	L5
Uses: Antineoplastic, anticancer drug	D

AAP: Not reviewed

T½= 2.6 hours; **RID=** ; **Oral** = Complete; **MW=** 246

Clinical: Busulfan is an alkylating agent used in chronic myeloid leukemia, and bone marrow transplant. See monograph in this book for more data. No data are available on the transfer of busulfan into human milk. However, approximately 20% enters the CNS, which suggest similar amounts could enter the milk compartment. Withhold breastfeeding for a minimum of 24 hours after use.

BUTABARBITAL; *Butisol, Butalan, Ampyrox*	L3
Uses: Sedative, hypnotic	D

AAP: Not reviewed

T½= 100 hours; **RID=** ; **Oral** = Complete; **MW=** 232

Clinical: Butabarbital is an old and weak barbiturate. We have little or no kinetic data on this product. Observe for sedation if this is routinely used. Avoid using this product in mothers with infants suffering from dyspnea or apnea, as barbiturates are potent inhibitors of the respiratory center. Other than apnea, the risks of using this product in breastfeeding mothers is probably minimal.

BUTALBITAL COMPOUND; *Fioricet, Fiorinal, Bancap, Two-Dyne, Tecnal, Fiorinal*	**L3**
Uses: Mild analgesic, sedative	**C**

AAP: Not reviewed

T½= 40-140 hours; **RID=** ; **Oral** = Complete; **MW=** 224

Clinical: We have no data on the transfer of butalbital into human milk, although transfer is likely due to its pharmacokinetic profile (low molecular weight, long half-life, low protein binding, distribution mainly in plasma). Butalbital is probably okay to use during breastfeeding. Observe for sedation in the breastfed infant.

BUTOCONAZOLE; *Gynezole-1*	**L3**
Uses: Anti-fungal	**C**

AAP: Not reviewed

T½= ; **RID=** ; **Oral** = ; **MW=** 474.8

Clinical: It is not known whether this drug is excreted in human milk. Because many drugs are excreted in human milk, caution should be exercised when butoconazole nitrate is administered to a nursing woman.

BUTORPHANOL; *Stadol*	**L2**
Uses: Potent narcotic analgesic	**C**

AAP: Maternal medication usually compatible with breastfeeding

T½= 4.56 hours; **RID=** 0.5%; **Oral** = 17 %; **MW=** 327

Clinical: Butorphanol levels in milk are quite low. The oral bioavailability is quite low. Taken together, these two points reduce the risk to a breastfeeding infant. Infants probably get much more in utero, than via milk.

CABERGOLINE; *Dostinex*	L4
Uses: Inhibits prolactin secretion	B

AAP: Not reviewed

T½= 63-69 hours;   **RID**= ;   **Oral** = Complete;   **MW**= 451

Clinical: Cabergoline is the preferred ergot alkaloid to suppress lactation. Milk levels are unreported. In cases where mothers have been erroniously treated early postpartum, they may be able to restart lactation with heavy pumping and breastfeeding. In cases of hyperprolactinemia, mothers may continue breastfeeding with lower or titrated doses of cabergoline.

CAFFEINE; *Vivarin, Nodoz, Coffee*	L2
Uses: CNS stimulant	C

AAP: Maternal medication usually compatible with breastfeeding

T½= 4.9 hours;   **RID**= 6% - 25.9%;   **Oral** = 100%;   **MW**= 194

Clinical: Caffeine during breastfeeding is probably safe. Observe for irritability and insomnia in the breastfed infant. Chronic intake of caffeine is not recommended during breastfeeding as it tends to accumulate in the infant's plasma in the neonatal period. There are some reports of reduced iron content in milk due to chronic caffeine intake.

CALCIPOTRIENE; *Dovonex, Taclonex Scalp*	L3
Uses: Synthetic Vitamin D3 used for treatment of psoriasis	C

AAP: Not reviewed

T½= ;   **RID**= ;   **Oral** = Variable;   **MW**= 430

Clinical: Only 5-6% is absorbed into the systemic circulation (via ointment). It is unlikely plasma levels of calcipotriene would be elevated at all, and milk levels would be virtually nil because vitamin D transport to milk is normally quite low. Calcipotriene is active however, and used over wide areas of the body could (but unlikely) lead to some absorption.

CALCITONIN; *Calcimar, Salmonine, Osteocalcin, Miacalcin, Caltine*	L3
Uses: Calcium metabolism	C

AAP: Not reviewed

T½= 43 minutes;   **RID**= ;   **Oral** = None;   **MW**=

Clinical: Calcitonin is unlikely to penetrate human milk due to its large molecular weight. Further, its oral bioavailability is nil due to destruction in the GI tract. It has been reported to inhibit lactation in animals although this has not been reported in humans.

CALCITRIOL; *Rocaltrol*	L3
Uses: Vitamin D analog	C

AAP: Not reviewed

T½= 5-8 hours; **RID=** ; **Oral** = Complete; **MW=** 416

Clinical: Vitamin D typically undergoes a series of metabolic steps to become active. Calcitriol (1,25 dihydro cholecalciferol) is believed to be the active metabolite of vitamin D metabolism. While plasma levels of vitamin D are normally quite low in human milk (<20 IU/L), at least one study now suggests that supplementing a mother with extraordinarily high levels of vitamin D2 can elevate milk levels, and subsequently could lead to hypercalcemia in a breastfed infant. See Vitamin D for new data.

CANDESARTAN; *Atacand, Amias*	L3
Uses: Antihypertensive agent	C

AAP: Not reviewed

T½= 9 hours; **RID=** ; **Oral** = 15%; **MW=** 611

Clinical: ACE inhibitors can be used in breastfeeding mothers postpartum without major risk in some cases with due caution. However, no data are available on candesartan in human milk although the manufacturer states that it is present in rodent milk and infants < 1 year of age should not be exposed to this drug. Some caution is recommended in the neonatal period and particularly when used in mothers with premature infants. Never use in pregnant women past the first trimester.

CANNABIS; *Marijuana, Tetrahydrocannabinol*	L5
Uses: Sedative, hallucinogen	C

AAP: Drugs of abuse for which adverse effects have been reported

T½= 25-57 hours; **RID=** ; **Oral** = 6-20%; **MW=** 314

Clinical: Marijuana has an enormous affinity for milk, with a milk/plasma ratio of 8. That said, the levels in milk are still low enough that clinical effects on infants appear unlikely. Thus far, studies suggest that the neurobehavioral outcome is normal. However, low levels of marijuana will appear in milk and inevitably in the infants urine for long periods following exposure. Infants will test urine-screen positive for marijuana residues for perhaps weeks after exposure.

CAPSAICIN; Zostrix, Axsain, Capsin, Capzasin-P, No-Pain, Absorbine Jr. Arthritis, ArthriCare, Qutenza	L3
Uses: Analgesic, topical	C

AAP: Not reviewed

T½= Several hours; **RID=** ; **Oral =** ; **MW=** 305

Clinical: No data is available on transfer into human milk. However, topical application to the nipple or areola should be avoided unless it is thoroughly removed prior to breastfeeding.

CAPTOPRIL; Capoten, Apo-Capto, Novo-Captopril	L2
Uses: Antihypertensive drug (ACE inhibitor)	C

AAP: Maternal medication usually compatible with breastfeeding

T½= 2.2 hours; **RID=** ; **Oral =** 60-75%; **MW=** 217

Clinical: In one report of 12 women treated with 100 mg three times daily, maternal serum levels averaged 713 µg/L while breast milk levels averaged 4.7 µg/L at 3.8 hours after administration. Data from this study suggest that an infant would ingest approximately 0.002% of the free captopril consumed by its mother (300mg) on a daily basis. No adverse effects have been reported in this study. Use with care in mothers with premature infants.

CARBAMAZEPINE; Tegretol, Epitol, Carbatrol, Apo-Carbamazepine, Mazepine	L2
Uses: Anticonvulsant	D

AAP: Maternal medication usually compatible with breastfeeding

T½= 18-54 hours; **RID=** 3.8% - 5.9%; **Oral =** 100%; **MW=** 236

Clinical: Infants of epileptic mothers treated with CBZ throughout pregnancy and breastfeeding should be carefully monitored for possible adverse effects. Watch for Drug-Drug Interactions. Probably safe to use in breastfeeding.

CARBAMIDE PEROXIDE; *Gly-Oxide, Debrox, Auro Otic, Teeth whiteners, Peroxides, Auro Ear Drops, Dewax*	L1
Uses: Antibacterial, whitening agent	C

AAP: Not reviewed

T½= ; **RID=** ; **Oral =** ; **MW=** 94

Clinical: This product is convered to hydrogen peroxide, which would never survive long enough in tissues to reach the milk compartment.

CARBENICILLIN; *Geopen, Geocillin, Carindacillin*	L1
Uses: Extended spectrum penicillin antibiotic	B

AAP: Not reviewed

T½= 1 hour; **RID=** 0.3%; **Oral =** <10-30%; **MW=** 378

Clinical: Only limited levels are secreted into breastmilk.   Due to its poor oral absorption (<10%) the amount absorbed by a nursing infant would be minimal.

CARBETAPENTANE; *Exhall, Expectuss*	L5
Uses: Cough suppressant	C

AAP: Not reviewed

T½= ; **RID=** ; **Oral =** ; **MW=**

Clinical: One report indicated that carbetapentane may be excreted in human milk in quantities large enough to cause respiratory problems in the infant.

CARBIDOPA; *Lodosyn, Sinemet*	L3
Uses: Inhibits levodopa metabolism	C

AAP: Not reviewed

T½= 1-2 hours; **RID=** ; **Oral =** 40-70%; **MW=** 244

Clinical: Use discretion in administering to pregnant or lactating women. Warning: Carbidopa and levodopa are known to suppress prolactin production in normal, and breastfeeding mothers.

CARBIMAZOLE	L3
Uses: Thyroid inhibitor	D

AAP: Maternal medication usually compatible with breastfeeding

T½= 6-13 hours; **RID=** 2.3% - 5.3%; **Oral =** Complete; **MW=** 186

Clinical: Carbimazole, a prodrug of methimazole, is rapidly and completely converted to the active methimazole in the plasma. Only methimazole is detected in plasma, urine and thyroid tissue. Milk levels of methimazole depend on maternal dose but appear too low to produce clinical effect.

CARBOPLATIN	L5
Uses: Anticancer	D

AAP: Not reviewed

T½= ; **RID=** 0.7% - 4.1%; **Oral =** ; **MW=**

Clinical: Very hazardous compound. No data are yet available on its transfer to milk. Breastfeeding is not recommended.

CARBOPROST TROMETHAMINE; *Hemabate*	L3
Uses: Oxytocic prostaglandin for postpartum hemorrhage	C

AAP: Not reviewed

T½= <1 hour; **RID=** ; **Oral =** ; **MW=** 489

Clinical: No data are available on its transfer to human milk. Prostaglandins have brief half-lives and little distribution out of the plasma compartment. It is not likely it will penetrate milk in clinically relevant amounts.

CARISOPRODOL; *Soma Compound, Solol, Soma*	L3
Uses: Muscle relaxant, CNS depressant	C

AAP: Not reviewed

T½= 8 hours; **RID=** 0.5% - 6.3%; **Oral =** Complete; **MW=** 260

Clinical: Carisoprodol is a commonly used skeletal muscle relaxant that is a CNS depressant. The average milk concentration of carisoprodol is 0.9 mg/L. No adverse effects on the infant were noted.

CARTEOLOL; *Cartrol*   L3

Uses: Beta-adrenergic antihypertensive   C

AAP: Not reviewed

T½= 6 hours; **RID=** ; **Oral =** 80%; **MW=** 292

Clinical: Carteolol is a typical beta-blocker used for hypertension. Carteolol is reported to be excreted in breastmilk of lactating animals. No data are available on levels in human milk.

CARVEDILOL; *Coreg, Eucardic, Proreg*   L3

Uses: Antihypertensive   C

AAP: Not reviewed

T½= 7-10 hours; **RID=** ; **Oral =** 25-35%; **MW=**

Clinical: There are no data available on the transfer of this drug into human milk. However, due to its high lipid solubility, some may transfer. As with any beta-blocker, some caution is recommended until milk levels are reported.

CASCARA SAGRADA; *Cascara Sagrada*   L3

Uses: Laxative   C

AAP: Maternal medication usually compatible with breastfeeding

T½= ; **RID=** ; **Oral =** ; **MW=**

Clinical: Trace amounts appear to be secreted into breastmilk. No exact estimates have been published. May cause loose stools and diarrhea in neonates.

CASPOFUNGIN ACETATE; *Cancidas*   L3

Uses: Antifungal   C

AAP: Not reviewed

T½= >11 hours; **RID=** ; **Oral =** Poor; **MW=** 1213

Clinical: No data are available for human milk. Regardless, the oral bioavailability is reported as poor and it is unlikely an infant would absorb enough to be clinically relevant, but this is only speculative.

CEFACLOR; *Ceclor, Apo-Cefaclor*   L1

Uses: Cephalosporin antibiotic   B

AAP:	Not reviewed

$T\frac{1}{2}$= 0.5-1 hr.; **RID**= 0.4% - 0.8%; **Oral** = 100%; **MW**= 386

Clinical: Commonly used pediatric cephalosporin antibiotic. Observe for changes in gut flora and diarrhea.

CEFADROXIL; *Ultracef, Duricef*	L1
Uses: Cephalosporin antibiotic	B

AAP: Maternal medication usually compatible with breastfeeding

$T\frac{1}{2}$= 1.5 hours; **RID**= 0.8% - 1.3%; **Oral** = 100%; **MW**= 381

Clinical: Cefadroxil is a typical first-generation, cephalosporin antibiotic. Small amounts are known to be secreted into milk. Observe for diarrhea.

CEFAZOLIN; *Ancef, Kefzol*	L1
Uses: Cephalosporin antibiotic	B

AAP: Maternal medication usually compatible with breastfeeding

$T\frac{1}{2}$= 1.2-2.2 hours; **RID**= 0.8%; **Oral** = Poor; **MW**= 455

Clinical: Cefazolin is a typical first-generation, cephalosporin antibiotic that has adult and pediatric indications. Cefazolin is poorly absorbed orally; therefore, the infant would absorb a minimal amount. Plasma levels in infants are reported to be too small to be detected.

CEFDINIR; *Omnicef*	L1
Uses: Antibiotic	B

AAP: Not reviewed

$T\frac{1}{2}$= 1.7 hours; **RID**= ; **Oral** = 21%; **MW**= 395

Clinical: Following administration of a 600 mg oral dose, no cefdinir was detected in human milk. As with other third generation cephalosporins, the use of this medication seems to be compatible with breastfeeding. Milk levels virtually undetectable. Observe for diarrhea.

CEFDITOREN; *Spectracef*	L2
Uses: Cephalosporin antibiotic	B

AAP: Not reviewed

T½= 1.3-2 hours; **RID=** ; **Oral =** 14%; **MW=** 620

Clinical: No data reported in breastfed infants. Observe for diarrhea.

CEFEPIME; *Maxipime*	L2
Uses: Cephalosporin antibiotic	B

AAP: Not reviewed

T½= 2 hours; **RID=** 0.3%; **Oral =** Poor; **MW=** 571

Clinical: Cefepime is secreted in human milk in small amounts averaging 0.5 mg/L. This amount is too small to produce any clinical symptoms other than possible changes in gut flora.

CEFIXIME; *Suprax*	L2
Uses: Cephalosporin antibiotic	B

AAP: Not reviewed

T½= 7 hours; **RID=** ; **Oral =** 30-50%; **MW=** 453

Clinical: Cefixime is an oral, third-generation cephalosporin used in treating infections. It is poorly absorbed by the oral route. It is secreted to a limited degree in the milk although in one study of a mother receiving 100 mg, it was undetected in the milk from 1-6 hours after the dose.

CEFOPERAZONE SODIUM; *Cefobid*	L2
Uses: Cephalosporin antibiotic	B

AAP: Not reviewed

T½= 2 hours; **RID=** 0.4% - 1%; **Oral =** Poor; **MW=** 645

Clinical: Cefoperazone is extremely acid labile and would be destroyed in the GI tract of an infant. It is unlikely that significant absorption would occur.

CEFOTAXIME; *Claforan*	L2
Uses: Cephalosporin antibiotic	B

AAP: Maternal medication usually compatible with breastfeeding

T½= 1 hour; **RID=** 0.3%; **Oral =** Poor; **MW=** 455

Clinical: Cefotaxime is poorly absorbed orally. Likely safe. Observe for GI symptoms such as diarrhea.

CEFOTETAN; *Cefotan*   L2

Uses: Cephalosporin antibiotic   B

AAP: Not reviewed

T½= 3-4.6 hours; **RID=** 0.2% - 0.3%; **Oral** = Poor; **MW=** 576

Clinical: Cefotetan is a third generation cephalosporin that is poorly
   absorbed orally and is only available via IM and IV injection.
   The drug is distributed into human milk in low concentrations.

CEFOXITIN; *Mefoxin*   L1

Uses: Cephalosporin antibiotic   B

AAP: Maternal medication usually compatible with breastfeeding

T½= 0.7-1.1 hour; **RID=** 0.1% - 0.3%; **Oral** = Poor; **MW=** 427

Clinical: Levels in milk are reportedly low. Observe for changes in
   gut flora.

CEFPODOXIME PROXETIL; *Vantin*   L2

Uses: Cephalosporin antibiotic   B

AAP: Not reviewed

T½= 2.09-2.84 hours; **RID=** ; **Oral** = 50%; **MW=** 558

Clinical: Only 50% is orally absorbed. Milk levels are low. Pediatric
   indications down to 6 months of age are available.

CEFPROZIL; *Cefzil*   L1

Uses: Oral cephalosporin antibiotic   B

AAP: Maternal medication usually compatible with breastfeeding

T½= 78 minutes; **RID=** 3.7%; **Oral** = Complete; **MW=**

Clinical: Levels in milk low. Probably safe for use in breastfeeding
   mothers. Observe for changes in gut flora. Pediatric indications
   for infants 6 months and older are available.

CEFTAZIDIME; *Ceftazidime, Fortaz, Tazidime, Ceptaz*   L1

Uses: Cephalosporin antibiotic   B

AAP: Maternal medication usually compatible with breastfeeding

T½= 1.4-2 hours; **RID=** 0.9%; **Oral** = <10%; **MW=** 547

Clinical: There is no progressive accumulation of ceftazidime in breastmilk, as evidenced by the similar levels prior to and after seven doses. The therapeutic dose for neonates is 30-50 mg/kg every 12 hours.

CEFTIBUTEN; *Cedax*	L2
Uses: Cephalosporin antibiotic	B

AAP: Not reviewed

T½= 2.4 hours; **RID=** ; **Oral** = High; **MW=** 410

Clinical: No data yet available on penetration into human breastmilk. Small to moderate amounts may penetrate into milk, ceftibuten is cleared for pediatric use.

CEFTIZOXIME; *Cefizox, Baxam*	L1
Uses: Cephalosporin antibiotic	B

AAP: Not reviewed

T½= 2.3 hours; **RID=** 0.3% - 0.6%; **Oral** = Minimal; **MW=** 383

Clinical: Breast milk levels in three studies are negligible. Observe for changes in gut flora. Of course, use with caution in infants allergic to cephalosporins.

CEFTRIAXONE; *Rocephin*	L1
Uses: Cephalosporin antibiotic	B

AAP: Maternal medication usually compatible with breastfeeding

T½= 7.3 hours; **RID=** 4.1% - 4.2%; **Oral** = Poor; **MW=** 555

Clinical: Ceftriaxone levels in breastmilk are probably too low to be clinically relevant, except for changes in GI flora. Ceftriaxone is commonly used in neonates.

CEFUROXIME; *Ceftin, Kefurox, Zinacef*	L2
Uses: Cephalosporin antibiotic	B

AAP: Not reviewed

T½= 1.4 hours; **RID=** 0.6% - 2%; **Oral** = 30-50%; **MW=** 424

Clinical: Cefuroxime is generally regarded as safe to use in breastfeeding, and transfer into milk is minimal. Observe the breastfed infant for diarrhea and rash. Poor oral bioavailability also lessens the effect on the breastfed infant.

CELECOXIB; *Celebrex*	L2
Uses: NSAID anti-inflammatory	C
AAP: Not reviewed	
T½= 11.2 hours; **RID**= 0.3% - 0.7%; **Oral** = 99%; **MW**= 381	
Clinical: Milk levels are reportedly quite low. Minimal risk to infants.	

CEPHALEXIN; *Keflex, Apo-Cephalex, Ceporex, Novo-Lexin*	L1
Uses: Cephalosporin antibiotic	B
AAP: Not reviewed	
T½= 50-80 minutes; **RID**= 0.5% - 1.5%; **Oral** = Complete; **MW**= 347	
Clinical: Observe for diarrhea in infants exposed to cephalexin in combination with probenecid. Probenecid would dramatically reduce clearance and thus increase plasma levels.	

CEPHALOTHIN; *Keflin, Ceporacin*	L1
Uses: Cephalosporin antibiotic	B
AAP: Not reviewed	
T½= 30-50 minutes; **RID**= 0.3% - 0.5%; **Oral** = Poor; **MW**= 396	
Clinical: Cephalothin is a cephalosporin antibiotic for use by IM or IV administration. Milk levels are minimal. Observe for changes in gut flora and diarrhea.	

CEPHAPIRIN; *Cefadyl*	L1
Uses: Cephalosporin antibiotic	B
AAP: Not reviewed	
T½= 24-36 minutes; **RID**= 0.3% - 0.4%; **Oral** = Poor; **MW**= 445	
Clinical: Cephapirin is a cephalosporin antibiotic for IM or IV administration. Milk levels are minimal. Observe for changes in gut flora.	

CEPHRADINE; *Velosef, Anspor*	L1
Uses: Cephalosporin antibiotic	B

AAP: Not reviewed

T½= 0.7-2 hours; **RID=** 0.3% - 0.5%; **Oral** = Complete; **MW=** 349

Clinical: Cephradine is typical first-generation cephalosporin antibiotic. Milk levels average about 0.6 mg/L. These levels are too low to be clinically relevant.

CETIRIZINE; *Zyrtec, Reactine*	L2
Uses: Antihistamine	B

AAP: Not reviewed

T½= 8.3 hours; **RID=** ; **Oral** = 70%; **MW=** 389

Clinical: Cetirizine is one of the preferred antihistamines during breastfeeding since it is non-sedating. Nevertheless, observe for sedation in the breastfed infant.

CEVIMELINE; *Evoxac*	L3
Uses: Treatment of dry mouth; Alzheimer's disease	C

AAP: Not reviewed

T½= 3-5 hours; **RID=** ; **Oral** = Complete; **MW=** 244

Clinical: Cholinergic agent. No data are available on its transfer into human milk. Due to its strong cholinergic effects, some caution is recommended in breastfeeding mothers. Observe closely for excess salivation, diarrhea, excess sweating, nausea, and urinary frequency and infection.

CHAMOMILE, GERMAN; *Hungarian Chamomile, Sweet False, Wild Chamomile*	L3
Uses: Anti-inflammatory, carminative	

AAP: Not reviewed

T½= ; **RID=** ; **Oral** = ; **MW=**

Clinical: Probably safe when used in limited amounts. German chamomile is reported to be uterotonic and teratogenic in rats, rabbits, and dogs although the dose of alpha-bisabolol used in these studies was excessively high. Some authors suggest this product should be avoided in pregnant and breastfeeding mothers, but the German Commission E considers it safe.

CHLORAL HYDRATE; *Aquachloral, Noctec, Nortec, Novo-Chlorhydrate*   L3

Uses: Sedative, hypnotic   C

AAP: Maternal medication usually compatible with breastfeeding

T½= 7-10 hours; **RID=** 2.6%; **Oral =** Complete; **MW=** 165

Clinical: Chloral hydrate is a sedative hypnotic. Small to moderate amounts are known to be secreted into milk. Mild drowsiness was reported in one infant. Infant growth and development were reported to be normal. Use with caution.

CHLORAMPHENICOL; *Chloromycetin, Ak-Chlor, Chloroptic, Sopamycetin*   L4

Uses: Antibiotic   C

AAP: Drugs whose effect on nursing infants is unknown but may be of concern

T½= 4 hours; **RID=** 3.2% - 8.5%; **Oral =** Complete; **MW=** 323

Clinical: Chloramphenicol is a broad-spectrum antibiotic. Milk levels are too low to produce overt toxicity in infants but could produce allergic sensitization to subsequent exposures. Generally, chloramphenicol is considered contraindicated in nursing mothers although it is occasionally used in infants. This antibiotic can be extremely toxic, particularly in newborns, and should not be used for trivial infections.

CHLORDIAZEPOXIDE; *Apo-Chlordiazepoxide, Librium, Libritabs, Solium, Apo-Chlordiazepoxide, Medilium*   L3

Uses: Antianxiety, benzodiazepine sedative   D

AAP: Not reviewed

T½= 5-30 hours; **RID=** ; **Oral =** Complete; **MW=** 300

Clinical: Chlordiazepoxide is an older benzodiazepine that belongs to Valium family. It is secreted in breastmilk in moderate but unreported levels. See Diazepam.

CHLORHEXIDINE; *Peridex, BactoShield, Betasept, Dyna-Hex, Hibiclens, Hibitane*   L4

Uses: Lozenge antimicrobial   B

AAP: Not reviewed

T½= <4 hours; **RID=** ; **Oral =** Poor; **MW=** 505

Clinical: Chlorhexidine should not be used directly on the nipple of breastfeeding mothers.

CHLOROQUINE; *Aralen, Novo-Chloroquine*	L2
Uses: Antimalarial	C

AAP: Maternal medication usually compatible with breastfeeding

T½= 72-120 hours; **RID=** 0.6% - 1.1%; **Oral** = Complete; **MW=** 320

Clinical: Data suggests that the transfer into milk is probably too low to affect an infant. Later studies suggest the relative infant dose of chloroqine and desethylchloroquin is about 2.3% and 1% respectively. Probably safe to use.

CHLOROTHIAZIDE; *Diuril*	L3
Uses: Diuretic	C

AAP: Maternal medication usually compatible with breastfeeding

T½= 1.5 hours; **RID=** 2.1%; **Oral** = 20%; **MW=** 296

Clinical: Chlorothiazide is a typical thiazide diuretic. Although thiazide diuretics are reported to produce thrombocytopenia in nursing infants, it is remote and unsubstantiated. Most thiazide diuretics are considered compatible with breastfeeding if doses are kept low and milk production is unaffected.

CHLORPHENIRAMINE; *Aller Chlor, Chlor-Tripolon, Chlor-Trimeton*	L3
Uses: Antihistamine	B

AAP: Not reviewed

T½= 12-43 hours; **RID=** ; **Oral** = 25-45%; **MW=** 275

Clinical: Chlorpheniramine is a commonly used antihistamine. Although no data are available on secretion into breastmilk, it has not been reported to produce side effects. Sedation is the only likely side effect. Use non-sedating antihistamines instead.

CHLORPROMAZINE; *Thorazine, Ormazine, Chlorpromanyl, Largactil, Novo-Chlorpromazine*	L3
Uses: Tranquilizer	C

AAP: Drugs whose effect on nursing infants is unknown but may be of concern

T½= 30 hours; **RID**= 0.3%; **Oral** = Complete; **MW**= 319

Clinical: Chlorpromazine is a powerful CNS tranquilizer. Small amounts are known to be secreted into milk. Chlorpromazine has a long half-life and is particularly sedating. Long-term use of this product in a lactating mother may be risky to the breastfed infant. There are consistent reports of this family of products increasing the risk of apnea and SIDS. Observer for sedation and lethargy and avoid if possible.

CHLORPROPAMIDE; *Diabinese, Apo-Chlorpropamide, Novopropamide*	L3
Uses: Oral hypoglycemic	C

AAP: Not reviewed

T½= 33 hours; **RID**= 10.5%; **Oral** = Complete; **MW**= 277

Clinical: Chlorpropamide stimulates the secretion of insulin in some patients. Milk levels reported to be approximately 5 mg/L of milk. This study lacked details and may not be accurate. May cause hypoglycemia in infant although effects are largely unknown and unreported.

CHLORPROTHIXENE; *Taractan, Tarasan*	L3
Uses: Sedative, tranquilizer	C

AAP: Drugs whose effect on nursing infants is unknown but may be of concern

T½= 8-12 hours; **RID**= 0.3%; **Oral** = <40%; **MW**= 316

Clinical: Sedative commonly used in psychotic or disturbed patients. Chlorprothixene is poorly absorbed orally (<40%) and has been found to increase serum prolactin levels in mothers. Although the milk/plasma ratios are relatively high, only modest levels of chlorprothixene are actually secreted into human milk.

CHLORTHALIDONE; *Thalitone*	L3
Uses: Diuretic	B

AAP: Not reviewed

T½= 40-60h; **RID**= ; **Oral** = ; **MW**= 338

Clinical: Thiazides are excreted in human milk. Because of the potential for serious adverse reactions in nursing infants from chlorthalidone, a decision should be made whether to discontinue nursing or to discontinue the drug, taking into account the importance of the drug to the mother.

CHOLERA VACCINE; *Cholera Vaccine, Dukoral*	L3
Uses: Cholera vaccination	C

AAP: Not reviewed

T½= ; RID= ; Oral = ; MW=

Clinical: Cholera vaccine is available in an oral preparation and a sterile injectable solution containing equal parts of phenol inactivated Ogawa and Inaba serotypes of Vibrio cholerae bacteria. Maternal immunization with cholera vaccine significantly increases levels of anti-cholera antibodies (IgA, IgG) in their milk. It is not contraindicated in nursing mothers. Breastfed infants are generally protected from cholera transmission. Immunization is approved from the age of 6 months and older.

CHOLESTYRAMINE; *Questran, Cholybar, Novo-Cholamine*	L1
Uses: Cholesterol binding resin	C

AAP: Not reviewed

T½= ; RID= ; Oral = 0%; MW=

Clinical: Cholestyramine is a bile salt chelating resin. It is not absorbed from the maternal GI tract. Therefore, it is not secreted into breastmilk.

CHONDROITIN SULFATE; *Viscoat*	L3
Uses: Biologic polymer used for arthritis	

AAP: Not reviewed

T½= ; RID= ; Oral = 0-13%; MW= 50,000

Clinical: Chondroitin is a biological polymer that acts as a flexible connecting matrix between the protein filaments in cartilage. Thus far, chondroitin has been found to be nontoxic. Its molecular weight averages 50,000 daltons, which is far too large to permit its entry into human milk. Combined with a poor oral bioavailability and large molecular weight, it is unlikely to pose a problem for a breastfed infant.

CHORIONIC GONADOTROPIN; *A.P.L., Chorex-5, Profasi, Gonic, Pregnyl, Novarel, Humegon Pregnyl, Profasi HP*	L3
Uses: Placental hormone	X

AAP: Not reviewed

T½= 5.6 hours; **RID**= ; **Oral** = 0%; **MW**= 47,000

Clinical: Human chorionic gonadotropin (HCG) is a large polypeptide hormone produced by the human placenta with functions similar to luteinizing hormone (LH). Due to the large molecular weight (47,000) of HCG, it would be extremely unlikely to penetrate into human milk. It is unabsorbed orally.

CHROMIUM; *Chromium Picrolinate*	L3
Uses: Metal supplement	C
AAP: Not reviewed	

T½= ; **RID**= ; **Oral** = <1%; **MW**= 52

Clinical: Trace metal, required in glucose metabolism. Less than 1% is absorbed following oral administration.

CICLESONIDE; *Omnaris*	L3
Uses: Corticosteroid	C
AAP: Not reviewed	

T½= 6-7 hours; **RID**= ; **Oral** = < 1%; **MW**= 540

Clinical: Ciclesonide is a topical corticosteroid used presently for allergic rhinitis. Ciclesonide and its metabolite, des-ciclesonide, have negligible oral bioavailability (< 1%) as it is poorly absorbed, and has a high first- pass absorption by the liver. While we have no data on its use in breastfeeding mothers, as with the other nasal steroids, this product poses little risk.

CICLOPIROX OLAMINE; *Loprox*	L3
Uses: Antifungal	B
AAP: Not reviewed	

T½= 1.7 hours; **RID**= ; **Oral** = ; **MW**= 268

Clinical: Ciclopirox is a broad-spectrum antifungal and is active in numerous species including tinea, candida albicans, and trichophyton rubrum. Topical application produces minimal systemic absorption; it is unlikely that topical use would expose the nursing infant to significant risks.

CIMETIDINE; *Tagamet, Apo-Cimetidine, Novo-Cimetine, Peptol*	L1
Uses: Reduces gastric acid production	B

AAP: Maternal medication usually compatible with breastfeeding

T½= 2 hours; **RID=** 9.8% - 32.6%; **Oral =** 60-70%; **MW=** 252

Clinical: Cimetidine transfers to milk in relatively high levels and seems to concentrate in milk, although no adverse effects are reported. Cimetidine is probably safe to use during breastfeeding since it is commonly used in pediatric patients at higher doses. The preferred Histamine-2 antagonist is famotidine since it is transferred minimally into milk. Proton pump inhibitors (omeprazole, lansoprazole, etc.) may also be a suitable alternatives.

CINNARIZINE	L3
Uses: Antiemetic	C

AAP: Not reviewed

T½= 3-6 hours; **RID=** ; **Oral =** ; **MW=** 368

Clinical: Cinnarizine is an antiemetic used for motion sickness, and is not available in the USA. No data are available on its use in breastfeeding mothers.

CIPROFLOXACIN; *Cipro, Ciloxan*	L3
Uses: Fluoroquinolone antibiotic	C

AAP: Maternal medication usually compatible with breastfeeding

T½= 4.1 hours; **RID=** 2.1% - 6.3%; **Oral =** 50-85%; **MW=** 331

Clinical: Ciprofloxacin is present in milk, although levels are low. Diarrhea and other gut complications could arise. Ophthalmic use is probably without complication.

CITALOPRAM; *Celexa*	L2
Uses: Antidepressant, SSRI	C

AAP: Not reviewed

T½= 36 hours; **RID=** 3.6%; **Oral =** 80%; **MW=** 405

Clinical: While the original anectdotal data suggested that symptoms such as somnolence, colic, restlessness may occur in breastfed infants exposed to citalopram, the majority of new data suggests these symptoms are minimal and may not be associated with therapy. All this newer data suggests that the risks of this product are probably quite low. However, recent data on escitalopram suggests it is a better alternative.

CLARITHROMYCIN; *Biaxin*	L1
Uses: Antibiotic	C

AAP: Not reviewed

T½= 5-7 hours; **RID**= 2.1%; **Oral** = 50%; **MW**= 748

Clinical: Clarithromycin transfer to milk is quite negligible. Only about 2% transfers, and this is unlikely to bother an infant. This antibiotic is commonly used in infants and children. Observe for diarrhea and thrush. This product is very bitter. No mention is made of this, but the taste of milk could be altered.

CLEMASTINE; *Tavist*	L4
Uses: Antihistamine	B

AAP: Drugs associated with significant side effects and should be given with caution

T½= 10-12 hours; **RID**= 5.2%; **Oral** = 100%; **MW**= 344

Clinical: Clemastine is a long-acting antihistamine. Reports in infants suggest drowsiness, refusal to feed. Do not use this antihistamine in breastfeeding mothers.

CLINDAMYCIN + TRETINOIN; *Cleocin, Veltin, Dalacin*	L2
Uses: Antibiotic	B

AAP: Maternal medication usually compatible with breastfeeding

T½= 2.4 hours; **RID**= 1% - 7.3%; **Oral** = 90%; **MW**= 425

Clinical: The dose of clindamycin in milk is negligible, less than 1-2 mg per day. This is unlikely to affect an infant. The risk of *C. Diffcle* overgrowth is low, as it is uncommon in infants. Topical use of clindamycin solutions in the mother is almost no risk at all. Maternal plasma levels of clindamycin are low to undetectable, milk levels would be even lower. Clindamycin is so commonly used in pediatric patients at high doses, the risk from clindamycin in breastmilk is miniscule.

CLINDAMYCIN TOPICAL	L3
Uses: Antibiotic	B

AAP: Not reviewed

T½= 2.4 hours; **RID**=; **Oral** = 90%; **MW**= 425

Clinical: Clindamycin applied topically is minimally absorbed. Use during breastfeeding poses minimal harm. Avoid application to the nipple. If MRSA is suspected on the nipple, treat orally.

CLINDAMYCIN VAGINAL; *Cleocin Vaginal, Dalacin Vaginal Cream*	L2
Uses: Antibiotic	B
AAP: Maternal medication usually compatible with breastfeeding	
T½= 2.9 hours; **RID=** ; **Oral** = 90%; **MW=** 425	
Clinical: Vaginal administration of clindamycin poses little to no threat to the breastfed infant. Absorption vaginally is exceedingly low, and transfer to breast milk is highly unlikely.	

CLOBAZAM; *Frisium*	L3
Uses: Benzodiazepine anxiolytic	C
AAP: Not reviewed	
T½= 17-31 hours; **RID=** ; **Oral** = 87%; **MW=** 301	
Clinical: Clobazam (Frisium) is a typical benzodiazepine very similar to Valium. As with diazepam (Valium), it could possibly reach elevated levels in a breastfeeding infant over time. No data are available on breastmilk concentrations.	

CLOBETASOL PROPIONATE; *Clobevate, Clobex, Cormax, Olux-E, Olux, Temovate E, Temovate, Taro-Clobetasol, Dermovate, Gen-Clobetasol, Novo-Clobetasol*	L5
Uses: Topical Corticosteroid	C
AAP: Not reviewed	
T½= ; **RID=** ; **Oral** = ; **MW=** 467	
Clinical: Due to the high potency of this steroid, do not use this product on the nipple or areola of a breastfeeding mother.	

CLOMIPHENE; *Clomid, Serophene, Milophene*	L3
Uses: Ovulation stimulator for ovulatory failure	X
AAP: Not reviewed	
T½= 5-7 days; **RID=** ; **Oral** = Complete; **MW=** 406	

Clinical: Clomiphene appears to be very effective in suppressing lactation when used up to 4 days postpartum. However, its efficacy in reducing milk production in women, months after lactation is established, is unknown but believed to be minimal. Use with caution in breastfeeding mothers.

CLOMIPRAMINE; *Anafranil, Apo-Clomipramine*	L2
Uses: Anti-obsessional, antidepressant drug	C

AAP: Drugs whose effect on nursing infants is unknown but may be of concern

T½= 19-37 hours; **RID=** 2.8%; **Oral** = Complete; **MW=** 315

Clinical: Clomipramine is a tricyclic antidepressant frequently used for obsessive-compulsive disorder. Levels in milk appear low. Plasma levels of clomipramine in the breastfed infants were below the limit of detection, suggesting minimal transfer to the infant via milk. No untoward effects were noted in any of the infants.

CLONAZEPAM; *Klonopin, Rivotril, Apo-Clonazepam, PMS-Clonazepam*	L3
Uses: Anticonvulsant, sedative	D

AAP: Not reviewed

T½= 18-50 hours; **RID=** 2.8%; **Oral** = Complete; **MW=** 316

Clinical: Transmission in milk is likely low. Although some reports of neurobehavioural complications exist, these are probably due to the fact the infant was exposed in utero over months, and then via milk, both of which probably contributed to higher levels. A suitable alternative is lorazepam.

CLONIDINE; *Catapres, Dixarit, Apo-Clonidine, Novo-Clonidine*	L3
Uses: Antihypertensive	C

AAP: Not reviewed

T½= 20-24 hours; **RID=** 0.9% - 7.1%; **Oral** = 75-100%; **MW=** 230

Clinical: Clonidine usage during breastfeeding may cause a decrease in prolactin secretion, which may decrease milk production early postpartum. There have been no reports of adverse effects, however observe for hypotension in the breastfed infant.

CLOPIDOGREL; *Plavix*	L3
Uses: Platelet aggregation inhibitor	B

AAP: Not reviewed

T½= 8 hours; **RID=** ; **Oral** = 50%; **MW=** 420

Clinical: Clopidogrel is only used in those patients who are aspirin-intolerant. It is not known if it transfers into human milk, but it does enter rodent milk.

CLORAZEPATE; *Tranxene, Tranxene-SD, Apo-Clorazepate, Novo-Clopate*	L3
Uses: Benzodiazepine sedative	D

AAP: Not reviewed

T½= 40-50 hours (metab); **RID=** ; **Oral** = 97%; **MW=** 408

Clinical: Clorazepate is a typical benzodiazepine. The primary metabolite, nordiazepam, is the same as from diazepam (Valium). Milk levels of nordiazepam are low.

CLOTRIMAZOLE; *Gyne-Lotrimin, Mycelex, Lotrimin, FemCare, Trivagizole, Canesten, Clotrimaderm, Myclo*	L1
Uses: Antifungal	B

AAP: Not reviewed

T½= 3.5-5 hours; **RID=** ; **Oral** = Poor; **MW=** 345

Clinical: Generally regarded as safe in breastfeeding. Topical and vaginal adminstration poses minimal risk. Oral administration of clotrimazole may pass into human milk, although we have no data available. However, clotrimazole has low oral absorption, and so the passage of clotrimazole through breast milk has low clinical relevance.

CLOXACILLIN; *Tegopen, Cloxapen, Apo-Cloxi, Novo-Cloxin, Orbenin*	L2
Uses: Penicillin antibiotic	B

AAP: Not reviewed

T½= 0.7-3 hours; **RID=** 0.4% - 0.8%; **Oral** = 37-60%; **MW=** 436

Clinical: Cloxacillin is an oral penicillin. As with most penicillins, it is unlikely these levels would be clinically relevant. Probably safe for use in breastfeeding mothers.

CLOZAPINE; *Clozaril*	L3
Uses: Antipsychotic, sedative	B

AAP: Drugs whose effect on nursing infants is unknown but may be of concern

T½= 8-12 hours; **RID=** 1.4%; **Oral =** 90%; **MW=** 327

Clinical: Clozapine is an atypical antipsychotic, sedative drug somewhat similar to the phenothiazine family. The change from day one to seven suggests that clozapine entry into mature milk is less. Caution.

CO-TRIMOXAZOLE; *TMP-SMZ, Bactrim, Cotrim, Septra, Novo-Trimel*	L3
Uses: Sulfonamide antibiotic	C

AAP: Maternal medication usually compatible with breastfeeding

T½= ; **RID=** ; **Oral =** ; **MW=**

Clinical: Co-trimoxazole is the mixture of trimethoprim and sulfamethoxazole. See individual monographs for each of these products. Probably quite safe.

COAL TAR; *Denorex, Neutrogena T/Gel, Pentrax, Tegrin, Zetar*	L2
Uses: Anti-psoriatic	C

AAP: Not reviewed

T½= ; **RID=** ; **Oral =** ; **MW=** 110

Clinical: None transferred into milk following large surface area use in breastfeeding mother. Infant was reported to have levels of pyrene metabolite probably due to skin to skin contact from mother to infant. Avoid contact of treated areas with infant.

COCAINE; *Crack*	L5
Uses: Powerful CNS stimulant, local anesthetic	C

AAP: Drugs of abuse for which adverse effects have been reported

T½= 0.8 hour; **RID=** ; **Oral =** Complete; **MW=** 303

Clinical: Cocaine is a local anesthetic and a powerful central nervous system stimulant. It is well absorbed from all locations including the stomach, nasal passages, intrapulmonary tissues via inhalation, and even via ophthalmic instillation. Adverse effects include agitation, nervousness, restlessness, euphoria, hallucinations, tremors, tonic-clonic seizures, and myocardial arrhythmias. Cocaine is definitely contraindicated in breastfeeding mothers.

CODEINE; *Empirin #3 # 4, Tylenol # 3 # 4, Paveral, Penntuss*	L3
Uses: Analgesic	C
AAP: Maternal medication usually compatible with breastfeeding	

T½= 2.9 hours; **RID=** 8.1%; **Oral =** Complete; **MW=** 299

Clinical: Low levels of codeine are secreted into milk, and low-moderate dosing of codeine is probably okay during breastfeeding. Apnea is the main concern. If the infant has a history of apnea or the mother is somnolent, caution is strongly advised. Observe for sedation, poor feeding, apnea, and constipation in the breastfed infant.

COENZYME Q10; *Ubiquinone, CoQ10, Ubidecarenone*	L3
Uses: Cofactor in electron transport chain	
AAP: Not reviewed	

T½= 34 hours; **RID=** ; **Oral =** Complete; **MW=** 863

Clinical: Coenzyme Q10 is a naturally occurring cofactor, it is generally synthesized within the cell. No data are available on ubiquinone levels in milk. Probably safe in breastfeeding mothers. But do not overdose.

COLCHICINE; *Colchicine, Colcrys*	L4
Uses: Analgesic in gouty arthritis	C
AAP: Maternal medication usually compatible with breastfeeding	

T½= 12-30 minutes; **RID=** 4.7% - 31.5%; **Oral =** Complete; **MW=** 399

Clinical: The use of colchicine in breastfeeding mothers is probably not advisable, as we have many other analgesics and anti-inflammatories that are superior for the treatment of gouty symptoms.

COLESEVELAM HCL; *WelChol*	**L1**
Uses: Cholesterol lower agent	**B**

AAP: Not reviewed

T½= ; **RID=** ; **Oral** = None; **MW=**

Clinical: Colesevelam is a non-absorbed, polymeric, lipid-lowering agent that prevents the absorption of bile acids from the intestines. The only potential problem of using this product in breastfeeding mothers is the lowering of maternal plasma cholesterol levels, and the possible lowering of milk cholesterol levels. Milk cholesterol is particularly important in infant neurodevelopment.

COLESTIPOL; *Colestid*	**L3**
Uses: Bile Acid Sequestrant	**C**

AAP: Not reviewed

T½= ; **RID=** ; **Oral** = 0%; **MW=** large

Clinical: Colestipol is a bile acid sequestrant that is used to inhibit absorption of cholesterol by binding to bile acid complexes and promoting excretion. Colestipol is almost totally unabsorbed from the GI tract and is unlikely to enter milk at all.

COMFREY; *Russian comfrey, Knitbone, Bruisewort, Blackwort, Slippery root*	**L5**
Uses: Herbal poultice	**X**

AAP: Not reviewed

T½= ; **RID=** ; **Oral** = Complete; **MW=**

Clinical: Comfrey has been claimed to heal gastric ulcers, hemorrhoids, and suppress bronchial congestion and inflammation. The product contains allantoin, tannin, and a group of dangerous pyrrolizidine alkaloids. Comfrey and members of this family are exceedingly dangerous and should not be used topically, ingested orally, or used in any form in breastfeeding or pregnant mothers.

CORTICOTROPIN; *ACT, Acthar, ACTH*	**L3**
Uses: Stimulates cortisol release	**C**

AAP: Not reviewed

T½= 15 minutes; **RID=** ; **Oral** = 0%; **MW=**

Clinical: ACTH is secreted by the anterior pituitary in the brain and stimulates the adrenal cortex to produce and secrete adrenocortical hormones (cortisol, hydrocortisone). As a peptide product, ACTH is easily destroyed in the infants' GI tract. None would be absorbed by the infant. Brief exposures are probably not contraindicated.

CROMOLYN SODIUM; *Nasalcrom, Gastrocrom, Intal, Nalcrom, Opticrom, Rhynacrom, Vistacrom*	**L1**
Uses: Antiasthmatic, antiallergic	**B**
AAP: Not reviewed	

$T\frac{1}{2}$= 80-90 minutes; **RID**= ; **Oral** = <1%; **MW**= 512

Clinical: Cromolyn sodium is probably safe to use during breastfeeding. There is minimal oral absorption (1%), and so it is highly unlikely to pass into human milk. There have been no harmful effects reported in breastfed infants.

CYCLAMATE	**L3**
Uses: Sweetener	
AAP: Not reviewed	

$T\frac{1}{2}$= ; **RID**= ; **Oral** = ; **MW**= 201

Clinical: Cyclamate is an artificial sweetener. Cyclamate is up to 50 times sweeter than sugar. There are no adequate and well-controlled studies or case reports in breastfeeding women.

CYCLOBENZAPRINE; *Flexeril, Cycoflex, Fexmid, Novo-Cycloprine*	**L3**
Uses: Muscle relaxant, CNS depressant	**B**
AAP: Not reviewed	

$T\frac{1}{2}$= 24-72 hours; **RID**= ; **Oral** = Complete; **MW**= 275

Clinical: We do not have data on transfer of cyclobenzaprine into milk, however transfer is probably similar to the tricyclic antidepressants, which is minimal. Cyclobenzaprine is probably okay to use during breastfeeding in lower doses. Metaxalone is a suitable alternative that we have more data on.

CYCLOPENTOLATE; *AK-Pentolate, Cyclogyl, Cylate, Ocu-Pentolate, Pentolair, Ak-Pentolate, Diopentolate, Minims Cyclopentolate*   **L3**

Uses: Anticholinergic for dilating pupils   **C**

AAP: Not reviewed

T½= 111 minutes; **RID=** ; **Oral =** ; **MW=**

Clinical: Cyclopentolate is use to dilate the pupils. It is a potent anticholinergic and some is absorbed systemically. Children and particularly infants would be extremely susceptible to this agent. While no data are available on the transfer of this agent into human milk, it is rather unlikely that significant quantities would enter as plasma levels are so low, and milk levels would be even lower. Some caution is recommended with this product. A waiting period of perhaps 6 hours following its use would be sufficient to reduce risks.

CYCLOPHOSPHAMIDE; *Neosar, Cytoxan, Cytoxan, Procytox*   **L5**

Uses: Antineoplastic   **D**

AAP: Cytotoxic drug that may interfere with cellular metabolism of the nursing infant

T½= 7.5 hours; **RID=** ; **Oral =** 75%; **MW=** 261

Clinical: No data are presently available. The kinetics of this agent are highly variable depending on renal function, creatinine clearance, liver function, etc. Waiting periods before returning to breastfeeding should be adjusted for this factor. Discontinue breastfeeding for a period of at least 72 hours.

CYCLOSERINE; *Seromycin*   **L3**

Uses: Anti-tuberculosis drug   **C**

AAP: Maternal medication usually compatible with breastfeeding

T½= 12+ hours; **RID=** 14.1%; **Oral =** 70-90%; **MW=** 102

Clinical: Cycloserine is an antibiotic primarily used for treating tuberculosis. It is a small molecule with a structure similar to the amino acid, D-alanine. Probably compatible with breastfeeding.

CYCLOSPORINE; *Sandimmune, Neoral, Restasis*   **L3**

Uses: Immunosuppressant   **C**

AAP: Cytotoxic drug that may interfere with cellular metabolism of the nursing infant

T½= 6-27 hours; **RID**= 0.4% - 3%; **Oral** = 28% pediatric; **MW**=

Clinical: At least 15 mother/infant pairs have been studied to date. Milk levels of cyclosporine have been reported to be uniformly low and the dose transferred to the infant subclinical and undetectable. However in one case the levels in the infant were near therapeutic. Thus it is reasonably safe to use this product in breastfeeding mothers as long as you occassionally monitor mother and infant for plasma levels of cyclosporine.

CYPROHEPTADINE; *Periactin, PMS-Cyproheptadine*	L3
Uses: Antihistamine	B

AAP: Not reviewed

T½= 16 hours; **RID**= ; **Oral** = ; **MW**= 287

Clinical: There are no data on cyproheptadine transfer to milk. The adverse effect to watch out for is sedation. Switching to a non-sedating antihistamine (loratadine, cetirizine) may be a suitable. alternative.

CYTARABINE; *Cytosar*	L5
Uses: Antineoplastic	D

AAP: Not reviewed

T½= 1-3 hours; **RID**= ; **Oral** = <20%; **MW**= 243

Clinical: Cytarabine is an antimetabolite used to treat various leukemias and lymphomas. No data has been reported on transfer into breastmilk. The compound is poorly absorbed orally and is therefore used IM or IV only. This drug would be extremely toxic to an infant and is generally contraindicated in breastfeeding mothers.

CYTOMEGALOVIRUS INFECTIONS; *Human Cytomegalovirus, CMV*	
Uses: Viral infection	C

AAP: Not reviewed

T½= ; **RID**= ; **Oral** = ; **MW**=

Clinical: Depending on the population, approximately 74% of mothers delivering premature infants are already CMV-seropositive and none of these infants have CMV isolated from their urine. Thus, if women (and fetus) are exposed prenatally, there is simply no risk at all of using the mothers milk. Earlier research suggested 25% of infants acquired CMV if their seropositive mothers' milk was not frozen prior to use. New data suggests that the seroconversion rate in the infants of seropositive mothers is about 5.7% and that the rate of CMV acquisition in premature infants fed their seronegative mothers milk or formula is zero to 11%. This new data suggests that the relative risk of using milk from seropositive mothers, whether frozen or fresh, is low.

DALTEPARIN SODIUM; *Fragmin, Low Molecular Weight Heparin*	L2
Uses: Anticoagulant	B

AAP: Not reviewed

T½= 2.3 hours; **RID=** ; **Oral** = None; **MW**= 4000

Clinical: Dalteparin is a low molecular weight polysaccharide fragment of heparin used clinically as an anticoagulant. Due to the polysaccharide nature of this product, oral absorption is unlikely. Further, because this study was done early postpartum, it is possible that the levels in 'mature' milk would be lower. The authors suggest that "it appears highly unlikely that puerperal thromboprophylaxis with LMWH has any clinically relevant effect on the nursing infant".

DANAZOL; *Danocrine, Cyclomen*	L5
Uses: Synthetic androgen, antigonadotropic agent	X

AAP: Not reviewed

T½= 4.5 hours; **RID=** ; **Oral** = Complete; **MW**= 337

Clinical: Danazol suppresses the pituitary-ovarian axis by inhibiting ovarian steroidogenesis resulting in decreased secretion of estradiol and may increase androgens. Danazol is believed to reduce plasma prolactin levels in individuals. Due to its effect on pituitary hormones and its androgenic effects, it may reduce the rate of breastmilk production although this has not been documented. No data on its transfer to human milk are available.

DANTROLENE; *Dantrium*	L4
Uses: Skeletal muscle relaxant	C

AAP: Not reviewed

T½= 8.7 hours; **RID=** 7.9%; **Oral =** 35%; **MW=** 314

Clinical: Pump and discard milk for 2 days following intravenous use of this product. Based on the elimination half-life (9.02 hours), the authors suggest that breastfeeding is safe 2 days after discontinuation of IV dantrolene administration in the mother. The infant should be monitored for nausea, vomiting, fatigue, and muscle weakness, which are all known side effects of therapeutic doses in adults.

DAPSONE; *Dapsone, Aczone, Avlosulfon*	**L4**
Uses: Sulfone antibiotic	**C**

AAP: Maternal medication usually compatible with breastfeeding

T½= 28 hours; **RID=** 6.3% - 22.5%; **Oral =** 86-100%; **MW=** 248

Clinical: This product is of some risk to an infant as the RID = 23% which is quite high. Mothers should probably not breastfeed if they are consuming dapsone orally. Topical application for acne is of minimal to no risk.

DAPTOMYCIN; *Cubicin*	**L1**
Uses: Antibiotic for resistant staphylococcus infections	**B**

AAP: Not reviewed

T½= 9 hours; **RID=** 0.1%; **Oral =** Unlikely; **MW=** 1620

Clinical: Reported levels in milk are quite low, only 44.7 ng/mL (C_{max}) and this would not be orally absorbed in the infant. After 4 weeks of exposure neither mom or infant reported adverse events.

DARBEPOETIN ALFA; *Aranesp*	**L3**
Uses: Colony stimulating factor	**C**

AAP: Not reviewed

T½= 21 hours; **RID=** ; **Oral =** Nil; **MW=** 37,000

Clinical: Molecular weight too large to enter milk and it would not be orally bioavailable. Probably of limited risk.

DARIFENACIN; *Enablex*	**L3**
Uses: Anticholinergic agent used for overactive bladder	**C**

AAP: Not reviewed

T½= 12.3 hours; **RID=** ; **Oral** = 15-19%; **MW=** 507

Clinical: Darifenacin is a potent anticholinergic. We do not yet have any data on this drug in breastfeeding mothers. Expect milk levels to be extremely low. That said, significant caution is still recommended with these agents as they could potentially produce significant anticholinergic symptoms in breastfed infants including dry mouth, delayed stomach emptying, constipation, urinary retention, etc.

DEET; *DEET, 6-12 Plus, Off!, Deep Woods Off!, Cutter Insect Repellent, Muskol, Diethyl-m-Toluamide, Diethyltoluamide*	L3
Uses: Insect repellant	

AAP: Not reviewed

T½= 2.5 hours; **RID=** ; **Oral** = Complete; 9-56% cutaneous; **MW=** 191

Clinical: DEET transfers through the skin significantly (5-17%), and produces plasma levels in users that are generally low. Small amounts of DEET probably do enter the milk compartment, but these are probably subclinical. Unfortunately, we do not have any studies of DEET levels in milk at this time. Plasma levels are virtually undetectable after 4 or more hours following a single use. Chronic use over many days could lead to significant absorption by the mother. Breastfeeding mothers should be advised to use this sparingly, use only on exposed skin surfaces, use lower concentrations (25% or less), and do not use repeatedly over many days, and do not apply directly to the breast or nipple.

DEFERASIROX; *Exjade*	L3
Uses: Iron chelating agent	B

AAP: Not reviewed

T½= 8-16 hours; **RID=** ; **Oral** = 70%; **MW=** 373

Clinical: There are no adequate and well- controlled studies in pregnant women. No data are available on the concentrations in the breast milk compartment, however it is unlikely that high concentrations would be in breast milk due to high protein binding. Should the mother breastfeed, the infant's ferritin and iron levels should be monitored. Modest oral iron supplementation in the infant would block absorption of any deferasirox.

DEFEROXAMINE; *Desferal, Desferrioxamine*	L3
Uses: Iron chelator	C

AAP: Not reviewed

T½= 3-6 hours; **RID=** ; **Oral =** Nil; **MW=** 656

Clinical: Deferoxamine is an iron-chelating agent. No data are available on its transfer into human milk, but it is very unlikely. Further, oral bioavailability of this product is virtually nil and it is not likely to harm a breastfeeding infant.

Dehydroepiandrosterone- DHEA	L3
Uses: Steroid	

AAP: Not reviewed

T½= ; **RID=** ; **Oral =** ; **MW=**

Clinical: DHEA is a metabolic precursor to testosterone and estrogen. The use of DHEA-S for labor induction has been associated with a decrease in milk production postpartum with no changes in prolactin levels. This may be due to the biotransformation of DHEA-S to estrogen.

DELAVIRDINE; *Rescriptor*	L3
Uses: Antiretroviral agent used in HIV infections	C

AAP: Not reviewed

T½= ; **RID=** ; **Oral =** ; **MW=**

Clinical: There are no adequate and well-controlled studies or case reports in breastfeeding women. Breastfeeding is not recommended in mothers who have HIV.

DESIPRAMINE; *Pertofrane, Norpramin, Novo-Desipramine*	L2
Uses: Tricyclic antidepressant	C

AAP: Drugs whose effect on nursing infants is unknown but may be of concern

T½= 7-60 hours; **RID=** 0.3% - 0.9%; **Oral =** 90%; **MW=** 266

Clinical: Desipramine is a tricyclic antidepressant. Levels in milk are generally very low. No untoward effects have been reported.

DESLORATADINE; *Clarinex*	L2
Uses: Antihistamine	C

AAP: Not reviewed

T½= 27 hours; **RID=** 0.03%; **Oral** = Good; **MW=** 310

Clinical: Desloratadine is the active metabolite of loratadine (Claritin) and its half-life is longer than the parent compound. While we do not have specific data on desloratadine, we do have a good report on the prodrug loratadine. Note, the AAP approves the use of loratadine in breastfeeding mothers. It has not yet reviewed desloratadine.

DESMOPRESSIN ACETATE; *DDAVP, Stimate, Rhinyle*	L2
Uses: Synthetic antidiuretic hormone	B

AAP: Not reviewed

T½= 75.5 minutes; **RID=** 0.08%; **Oral** = 0.16%; **MW=** 1069

Clinical: Desmopressin (DDAVP) is a small synthetic octapeptide antidiuretic hormone. This peptide has been used in lactating women without effect on nursing infants.

Because DDAVP is easily destroyed in the gastrointestinal tract by trypsin, the oral absorption of these levels in milk would be nil.

DESOGESTREL + ETHINYL ESTRADIOL; *Mircette, Cyclessa*	L3
Uses: Low dose oral contraceptive	X

AAP: Not reviewed

T½= ; **RID=** ; **Oral** = ; **MW=**

Clinical: Mircette is a somewhat atypical lower-dose estrogen/progestin oral contraceptive. Estrogen-containing contraceptives may interfere with milk production by decreasing the quantity and quality of milk production.

DESVENLAFAXINE; *Pristiq*	L3
Uses: Antidepressant, SSRI, SSNRI	C

AAP: Not reviewed

T½= 11 hours; **RID=** 6.8% - 9.3%; **Oral** = 80%; **MW=** 263

Clinical: Desvenlafaxine is an active metabolite of venlafaxine with similar antidepressant activity. While no data are available on the transmission of this product specifically into human milk, we do have excellent data on the transmission of desvenlafaxine into human milk following the use of its precursor, venlafaxine. See venlafaxine.

DEXAMETHASONE; *Decadron, AK-Dex, Maxidex*	L3
Uses: Corticosteroid anti-inflammatory	C
AAP: Not reviewed	
T½= 3.3 hours; **RID**= ; **Oral** = 78%; **MW**= 392	

Clinical: There is little harm in taking dexamethasone while breastfeeding, unless it is used at high doses for prolonged periods of time. We have no data on its transfer into milk; it is probably similar to prednisone levels in milk which are low. Observe for impaired bone growth and GI ulcers, however no adverse effects have been reported in the breastfed infant.

DEXBROMPHENIRAMINE; *Drixoral*	L3
Uses: Antihistamine	
AAP: Not reviewed	
T½= 25 hours; **RID**= ; **Oral** = well absorbed; **MW**=	

Clinical: Dexbrompheniramine is a first-generation antihistamine with anticholinergic properties. One case report of a 3-month old nursing infant suggests that it causes irritability, excessive crying, and difficulty sleeping; symptoms resolved after discontinuation of dexbrompheniramine 6 mg.

DEXLANSOPRAZOLE; *Kapidex*	L2
Uses: Suppresses gastric acid secretion	B
AAP: Not reviewed	
T½= 1-2 hours; **RID**= ; **Oral** = Poor; **MW**= 369	

Clinical: Dexlansoprazole is a new proton pump inhibitor and is the active metabolite of lansoprazole (Prevacid). Structurally similar to omeprazole and lansoprazole, it is very unstable in stomach acid and to a large degree would be largely denatured by acidity of the infant's stomach

DEXMETHYLPHENIDATE; *Focalin*   **L3**

Uses: CNS stimulant, treatment of ADHD   **C**

AAP: Not reviewed

T½= 2-4.5 hours for immediate release; **RID=** ; **Oral** = 22-25%; **MW=** 270

Clinical: Dexmethylphenidate is a CNS stimulant that is used mainly in the treatment of ADHD. It is not known whether dexmethylphenidate is excreted in human milk.

DEXTROAMPHETAMINE; *Dexedrine, Amphetamine, Oxydess, Adderall, Vyvanse, Adderall XR*   **L3**

Uses: Powerful CNS stimulant   **C**

AAP: Drugs of abuse for which adverse effects have been reported

T½= 6-8 hours; **RID=** 1.8% - 6.9%; **Oral** = Complete; **MW=** 368

Clinical: Dextroamphetamine apparently transfers into milk avidly. Of the 6 infants studied thus far, no untoward effects have been reported in any infant. If this product is used in breastfeeding mothers, the dose should be kept low, and infants should be monitored for agitation, and poor weight gain. Methylphenidate is probably preferred.

DEXTROMETHORPHAN; *DM, Benylin, Delsym, Pertussin, Robitussin DM, Balminil-DM, Delsym, Benylin DM*   **L1**

Uses: Antitussive, Cough preparation   **C**

AAP: Not reviewed

T½= <4 hours; **RID=** ; **Oral** = Complete; **MW=** 271

Clinical: Dextromethorphan is a weak antitussive commonly used in infants and adults. It is the safest of the antitussives and is routinely used in children and infants. No data on its transfer to human milk are available. It is very unlikely that enough would transfer via milk to provide clinically significant levels in a breastfed infant.

DIAZEPAM; *Valium, Apo-Diazepam, Meval, Novo-Dipam, Vivol*   **L3**

Uses: Sedative, anxiolytic drug   **D**

AAP: Drugs whose effect on nursing infants is unknown but may be of concern

T½= 43 hours; **RID**= 7.1%; **Oral** = Complete; **MW**= 285

Clinical: Diazepam is probably okay to use during breastfeeding. Observe for sedation, poor suckling, lethargy, withdrawal in the breastfed infant. The preferred benzodiazepines in breastfeeding are lorazepam and alprazolam.

DIBUCAINE; *Nupercainal, Cinchocaine*	L3
Uses: Local anesthetic	C
AAP: Not reviewed	

T½= ; **RID**= ; **Oral** = ; **MW**= 379

Clinical: Dibucaine is a long-acting local anesthetic generally used topically. No data are available on transfer to breastmilk. It is probably compatible with breastfeeding if use over small areas of the skin.

DICLOFENAC; *Cataflam, Voltaren, Pennsaid, Apo-Diclo, Novo-Difenac*	L2
Uses: NSAID analgesic for arthritis	C
AAP: Not reviewed	

T½= 1.1 hours; **RID**= ; **Oral** = Complete; **MW**= 318

Clinical: Diclofenac is a typical nonsteroidal analgesic (NSAID). Reported levels in milk are probably far too low to affect an infant.

DICLOXACILLIN; *Pathocil, Dycill, Dynapen*	L1
Uses: Penicillin antibiotic	B
AAP: Not reviewed	

T½= 0.6-0.8 hour; **RID**= 0.6% - 1.4%; **Oral** = 35-76%; **MW**= 470

Clinical: Transfer of dicloxacillin into human milk is minimal, and it is considered safe to use during breastfeeding. Adverse effects include diarrhea and candida diaper rash in the infant. This drug is the most commonly prescribed drug for treating mastitis in breastfeeding mothers.

DICYCLOMINE; *Bentyl, Antispas, Spasmoject, Bentylol, Formulex, Lomine*	L4
Uses: Anticholinergic, drying agent	B

AAP: Not reviewed

T½= 9-10 hours; **RID**= 6.9%; **Oral** = 67%; **MW**= 345

Clinical: Following a dose of 20 mg in a lactating woman, a 12-day-old infant reported severe apnea. Do not use in breastfeeding women.

DIDANOSINE; *Videx*	L3
Uses: Antiretroviral agent used in HIV infections	B

AAP: Not reviewed

T½= ; **RID**= ; **Oral** = ; **MW**=

Clinical: There are no adequate and well-controlled studies or case reports in breastfeeding women. Breastfeeding is not recommended in mothers who have HIV.

DIENOGEST and ESTRADIOL VALERATE; *Natazia*	L3
Uses: Oral contraceptive	

AAP: Not reviewed

T½= ; **RID**= ; **Oral** = ; **MW**=

Clinical: Estrogen-containing birth control preparations should be avoided in breastfeeding mothers due to reductions in milk production.

DIETHYLPROPION; *Tepanil, Tenuate, Tenuate*	L5
Uses: Anorexiant	B

AAP: Not reviewed

T½= 8 hours; **RID**= ; **Oral** = 70%; **MW**= 205

Clinical: Diethylpropion belongs to the amphetamine family and is typically used to reduce food intake. No data available other than manufacturer states this medication is secreted into breastmilk. The use of this medication during lactation is simply unrealistic and not justified.

DIETHYLSTILBESTROL; *Honvol*	L5
Uses: Synthetic estrogen	X

AAP: Not reviewed

T½= ; **RID**= ; **Oral** = Complete; **MW**= 268

Clinical: Diethylstilbestrol is known to produce a high risk of cervical cancer in female infants exposed during pregnancy. Do not use this estrogen during breastfeeding. Contraindicated.

DIFLUNISAL; *Dolobid, Apo-Diflunisal, Novo-Diflunisal*	**L3**
Uses: Nonsteroidal antiinflammatory analgesic	**C**

AAP: Not reviewed

T½= 8-12 hours; **RID**= 7.8% - 11.5%; **Oral** = Complete; **MW**= 250

Clinical: Diflunisal is excreted into human milk in concentrations 2-7% of the maternal plasma levels. This product is potentially a higher risk NSAID and other less toxic compounds should be used.

DIGOXIN; *Lanoxin, Lanoxicaps, Novo-Digoxin*	**L2**
Uses: Cardiac stimulant	**C**

AAP: Maternal medication usually compatible with breastfeeding

T½= 39 hours; **RID**= 2.7% - 2.8%; **Oral** = 65-85%; **MW**= 781

Clinical: Digoxin levels in milk are low. Plasma levels in the infants were undetectable.

DILTIAZEM HCL; *Cardizem SR, Dilacor-XR, Cardizem CD, Cartia XT, Cardizem, Apo-Diltiazem, Apo-Diltiaz*	**L3**
Uses: Antihypertensive, calcium channel blocker	**C**

AAP: Maternal medication usually compatible with breastfeeding

T½= 3.5-6 hours; **RID**= 0.9%; **Oral** = 40-60%; **MW**= 433

Clinical: Levels in milk are generally low. While nifedipine is probably a preferred choice calcium channel blocker because of our experience with it, the relative infant dose with this agent is quite small and it is not likely to be problematic.

DIMENHYDRINATE; *Marmine, Dramamine, Gravol, Traveltabs*	**L2**
Uses: Antihistamine for vertigo and motion sickness	**B**

AAP: Not reviewed

T½= 8.5 hours; **RID**= ; **Oral** = ; **MW**= 470

Clinical: The active constituent diphenhydramine is probably safe to use during breastfeeding. Observe for sedation in the breastfed infant. Suitable alternative antihistamines that are non-sedating are loratadine and cetirizine.

DIMETHYLSULFOXIDE; *DMSO, Rimso-50, DMSO2, MSM*	L3
Uses: Solvent used for arthritis, etc.	C

AAP: Not reviewed

T½= 11-14 hours (dermal); RID= ; Oral = Complete; MW=

Clinical: There are no adequate and well- controlled studies in pregnant women. While DMSO is relatively nontoxic,   it penetrates to many compartments and it would probably penetrate into milk in significant quantities. Due to the high plasma levels above, it is probable that milk levels would be quite high as well. Although the overall toxicity of this compound is quite minimal, exposing an infant to this agent, which is minimally efficacious, is probably not justified.

DINOPROSTONE; *Prostin E2, Prepidil, Cervidil*	L3
Uses: Prostaglandin E-2	C

AAP: Not reviewed

T½= 2.5-5 minutes; RID= ; Oral = ; MW=

Clinical: Dinoprostone is a naturally occurring prostaglandin E2 that is primarily used for induction of labor, for cervical ripening, as an abortifacient, for postpartum bleeding, and for uterine atony. The amount of dinoprostone entering milk is not known, but a brief wash out period would preclude any possible side effects.

DIPHENHYDRAMINE; *Benadryl, Cheracol, Allerdryl, Insomnal, Nytol*	L2
Uses: Antihistamine, antitussive	B

AAP: Not reviewed

T½= 4.3 hours; RID= 0.7% - 1.4%; Oral = 43-61%; MW= 255

Clinical: Diphenhydramine is probably safe to use during breastfeeding. Observe for sedation in the breastfed infant. Suitable alternative antihistamines that are non-sedating include loratadine and cetirizine.

DIPHENOXYLATE; *Lomotil, Lofene* | L3

Uses: Antidiarrheal	C

AAP: Not reviewed

T½= 2.5 hours; **RID=** ; **Oral =** 90%; **MW=** 453

Clinical: Diphenoxylate belongs to the opiate family and acts on the intestinal tract inhibiting GI motility and excessive GI propulsion. Although no reports on its transfer to human milk are available, it is probably secreted in breastmilk in very small quantities.

DIPHTHERIA AND TETANUS TOXOID; *DT, Td* | L3

Uses: Vaccine	C

AAP: Not reviewed

T½= ; **RID=** ; **Oral =** ; **MW=**

Clinical: Diphtheria and tetanus toxoid contains large molecular weight protein toxoids. It is extremely unlikely proteins of this size would be secreted in breastmilk. No data are available on its transfer to human milk.

DIPHTHERIA-TETANUS-PERTUSSIS; *DTaP, Acel-Imune, Tripedia, Tetramune, DPT* | L2

Uses: Vaccine	B

AAP: Not reviewed

T½= ; **RID=** ; **Oral =** ; **MW=**

Clinical: DTAP vaccine is safe for use in infants. TDAP for mothers is also safe to use. Both are inactivated vaccines, which pose minimal risk. No adverse effects have been reported in breastfed infants.

DIPIVEFRIN; *AK-Pro, Propine, PSM-Dipivefrin* | L2

Uses: Adrenergic for glaucoma	B

AAP: Not reviewed

T½= ; **RID=** ; **Oral =** Minimal; **MW=**

Clinical: Dipivefrin is a synthetic amine prodrug that is metabolized to epinephrine. It is not known if dipivefrin enters milk, but small amounts may be present. It is unlikely that any dipivefrin or epinephrine present in milk would be orally bioavailable to the infant.

DIPYRIDAMOLE; *Persantine, Apo-Dipyridamole, Novo-Dipiradol*	L3
Uses: Vasodilator, antiplatelet agent	B

AAP: Not reviewed

T½= 10-12 hours; **RID**= ; **Oral** = Poor; **MW**= 505

Clinical: According to the manufacturer, only small amounts are believed to be secreted in human milk. No reported untoward effects have been reported.

DIRITHROMYCIN; *Dynabac*	L3
Uses: Macrolide antibiotic	C

AAP: Not reviewed

T½= 20-50 hours; **RID**= ; **Oral** = 6-14%; **MW**=

Clinical: Dirithromycin is a macrolide antibiotic similar to the erythromycins. No data on the transfer of erythromycyclamine into human milk is available.

DISOPYRAMIDE; *Norpace, Napamide, Rythmodan*	L2
Uses: Antiarrhythmic	C

AAP: Maternal medication usually compatible with breastfeeding

T½= 8.3-11.65 hours; **RID**= 3.4%; **Oral** = 60-83%; **MW**= 339

Clinical: Disopyramide is secreted into milk in low levels. Such levels are probably too small to affect an infant. No side effects were reported.

DISULFIRAM; *Antabuse*	L5
Uses: Inhibitor of alcohol metabolism	C

AAP: Not reviewed

T½= ; **RID**= ; **Oral** = 80-90%; **MW**= 296

Clinical: The consumption of only minimal amounts of alcohol (cough syrup, nose drops, etc) could cause severe reactions in an infant. Mothers should not consume this potent drug.

DOCOSAHEXAENOIC ACID (DHA) | L3

Uses: Unsaturated oil

AAP: Not reviewed

T½= 20 hours; **RID**= ; **Oral** = ; **MW**= 328.488

Clinical: Unsaturated oil. Probably safe. Milk levels are relatively high. Use moderate doses.

DOCUSATE; *Colace, Docusate, Softgels, Dialose, Surfak, Albert Docusate, Colax-C, Colace, Surfak* | L2

Uses: Laxative, stool softener | C

AAP: Not reviewed

T½= ; **RID**= ; **Oral** = Poor; **MW**= 444

Clinical: Docusate is a detergent commonly used as a stool softener. Although some drug is absorbed by mother via her GI tract, transfer into breastmilk is unknown but probably minimal. Watch for loose stools in infant. It is not likely this would be overly detrimental to a breastfed infant.

DOLASETRON MESYLATE; *Anzemet* | L3

Uses: Antinauseant and antiemetic | B

AAP: Not reviewed

T½= 8.1 hours; **RID**= ; **Oral** = 75%; **MW**= 438

Clinical: No data are available on its transfer to milk. The maximum concentration in maternal plasma would be 556 ng/mL, which is quite low. At this plasma level, an infant would likely receive far less than a milligram daily. It has been safely used in children 2 years of age at doses of 1.2 mg/kg.

DOMPERIDONE; *Motilium, Motilidone* | L1

Uses: Gastrokinetic agent, galactagogue | C

AAP: Maternal medication usually compatible with breastfeeding

T½= 7-14 hours; **RID**= 0.01% - 0.04%; **Oral** = 13-17%; **MW**= 426

Clinical: Domperidone (Motilium) is a peripheral dopamine antagonist (similar to Reglan) generally used for controlling nausea and vomiting, dyspepsia, and gastric reflux. It differs from metoclopramide, in that domperidone does not enter the blood brain barrier, hence it has limited CNS activity such as extrapyramidal symptoms, depression, or stroke as with metoclopramide. While the FDA has issued a warning on this product, there is no good evidence that its use orally in doses of 10-20 three to four times daily produces arrhythmias. It's milk levels are many times lower than with metoclopramide, and its' oral bioavailability is poor (<13-17%). Doses in the 10 mg range produce significant increases in serum prolactin, and hence stimulate milk production.

DONEPEZIL; *Aricept*	L3
Uses: Cholinesterase inhibitor in Alzheimer's disease	C
AAP: Not reviewed	
T½= 70 hours; **RID=** ; **Oral** = 100%; **MW=** 415	

Clinical: No data are available on its transfer to human milk. Due to its long half-life, and its ability to affect cholinergic function in all mammals, some caution is recommended in breastfeeding women until data is available.

DOPAMINE-DOBUTAMINE; *Intropin, Revimine--Dobutrex*	L2
Uses: Adrenergic stimulants	C
AAP: Not reviewed	
T½= 2 minutes; **RID=** ; **Oral** = Poor; **MW=** 153	

Clinical: Dopamine and dobutamine are catecholamine pressor agents used in shock and severe hypotension. They are rapidly destroyed in the GI tract and are only used IV. It is not known if they transfer into human milk, but the half-life is so short they would not last long. Dopamine, while in the plasma, significantly (>60%) inhibits prolactin secretion and would likely inhibit lactation while being used.

DORIPENEM; *Doribax*	L3
Uses: Antibiotic	B
AAP: Not reviewed	
T½= 1 hour; **RID=** ; **Oral** = Poor; **MW=** 438	

Clinical: Doripenem is a new carbapenem antibiotic similar in structure to the penecillins. No data are available on its use in breastfeeding mothers, but levels in milk will likely be low, and the oral bioavailability in infants low as well. Observe for diarrhea and changes in gut flora.

DORNASE; *Pulmozyme*	L2
Uses: Mucolytic enzyme	B

AAP: Not reviewed

T½= ; **RID=** ; **Oral** = None; **MW=**

Clinical: Dornase is a mucolytic enzyme used in the treatment of cystic fibrosis. It is a large molecular weight peptide. It is poorly absorbed by the pulmonary tissues. Serum levels are undetectable. Even if it were to reach the milk, it would not be orally bioavailable in the infant.

DORZOLAMIDE; *Trusopt*	L3
Uses: Carbonic anhydrase inhibitor for open-angle glaucoma	C

AAP: Not reviewed

T½= ; **RID=** ; **Oral** = ; **MW=** 361

Clinical: Dorzolamide binds to RBC carbonic anhydrase(CA) for long periods (T½= 147 days) and reduces the CA activity in the RBC by as much as 50%. Dorzolamide is a carbonic anhydrase inhibitor used to treat ocular hypertension, open-angle glaucoma, etc. We do not have data on transfer to milk, but because plasma levels are incredibly low, levels in milk are probably low to undetectable. Do not use in mothers with infants who have poor creatinine clearance, such as premature infants. Risk level with this product is probably quite low.

DOTHIEPIN; *Prothiaden*	L2
Uses: Tricyclic antidepressant	D

AAP: Drugs whose effect on nursing infants is unknown but may be of concern

T½= 14.4-23.9 hours; **RID=** 0.8% - 2.2%; **Oral** = 30%; **MW=** 295

Clinical: This is a new analog of the older tricyclic antidepressant amitriptyline. Dothiepin appears in breastmilk in a concentration of 11 µg/L following a dose of 75 mg/day. In an outcome study of 15 mother/infant pairs 3-5 years postpartum, no overall cognitive differences were noted in dothiepin treated mothers/infants, suggesting that this medication did not alter cognitive abilities in breastfed infants.

DOXAZOSIN MESYLATE; *Cardura*	L4
Uses: Antiadrenergic antihypertensive	C

AAP: Not reviewed

T½ = 9-22 hours; **RID** = ; **Oral** = 62-69%; **MW** = 451

Clinical: Studies in lactating animals indicate milk levels that are 20 times that of maternal plasma levels, suggesting a concentrating mechanism in breastmilk. It is not known if this occurs in human milk. Extreme caution recommended.

DOXEPIN CREAM; *Zonalon cream, Zonalon*	L4
Uses: Antipruritic cream	B

AAP: Drugs whose effect on nursing infants is unknown but may be of concern

T½ = 28-52 hours; **RID** = ; **Oral** = Complete; **MW** = 279

Clinical: Doxepin cream is an antihistamine-like cream used to treat severe itching. Small but significant amounts are secreted in milk. Two published reports indicate absorption by infant varying from significant to modest but only in mother consuming oral doses. Caution.

DOXEPIN; *Adapin, Sinequan, Silenor, Triadapin, Novo-Doxepin*	L5
Uses: Antidepressant	C

AAP: Drugs whose effect on nursing infants is unknown but may be of concern

T½ = 8-24 hours; **RID** = 1.2% - 3%; **Oral** = Complete; **MW** = 279

Clinical: Small but significant amounts are secreted in milk. Two published reports indicate absorption by infant varying from significant to modest. Although the milk concentrations were low, the infant's plasma level of metabolite was similar to the maternal plasma level. It is apparent that the active metabolite of doxepin can concentrate in nursing infants and may be hazardous. We have numerous other antidepressants that are much safer and are preferred in breastfeeding mothers.

DOXERCALCIFEROL; *Hectorol, Hectoral*	**L3**
Uses: Vitamin D analog	**B**
AAP: Not reviewed	

T½= 32-37 hours; **RID=** ; **Oral =** Complete; **MW=**

Clinical: Doxercalciferol is a vitamin D analog indicated for the treatment of hyperparathyroidism. Excessive doses may lead to dangerously elevated plasma calcium levels. No data are available on its transfer into human milk. It is not likely that normal doses would lead to clinically relevant levels in human milk, particularly since vitamin D transfers only minimally into human milk. Some caution with these highly active forms of vitamin D is recommended.

DOXORUBICIN; *Adriamycin*	**L5**
Uses: Anticancer drug	**D**
AAP: Cytotoxic drug that may interfere with cellular metabolism of the nursing infant	

T½= 24-36 hours; **RID=** ; **Oral =** Poor; **MW=** 544

Clinical: Significant amounts of doxorubicin are transferred into human milk, and the half-life is very long. Doxorubicin is contraindicated in breastfeeding. Extremely toxic to breastfeeding infants, use is not recommended. Because this product is detectable in plasma (and milk) for long periods, a waiting period of approximately 7-10 days is recommended.

DOXYCYCLINE; *Doxychel, Vibramycin, Periostat,* *Apo-Doxy, Doxycin, Vibramycin, Vibra-Tabs, Doryx*	**L3**
Uses: Tetracycline antibiotic	**D**
AAP: Not reviewed	

T½= 15-25 hours; **RID**= 4.2% - 13.3%; **Oral** = 90-100%; **MW**= 462

Clinical: It is well-known that tetracyclines as a class tend to stain the teeth yellow after prolonged exposure. Doxycycline is the least staining of the tetracyclines, and short-term usage should be fine. Prolonged exposure may lead to impaired bone growth and increased likelihood of staining. Treatment for up to 3 weeks is acceptable in breastfeeding mothers.

DOXYLAMINE; *Unisom Nighttime*	L3
Uses: Antihistamine, sedative.	A
AAP: Not reviewed	

T½= 10.1 hours; **RID**= ; **Oral** = Complete; **MW**= 270

Clinical: Doxylamine is an antihistamine similar in structure to Benadryl. Because it has strong sedative properties, it is primarily used in over-the-counter sleep aids. Like other such antihistamines, it should be used only cautiously in infants and particularly in premature or term neonates due to paradoxical effects such as CNS stimulation or even sedation. Levels in breastmilk are not known but caution is recommended particularly in infants with apnea or other respiratory syndromes.

DROPERIDOL; *Inapsine*	L3
Uses: Tranquilizer, antiemetic	C
AAP: Not reviewed	

T½= 2.2 hours; **RID**= ; **Oral** = ; **MW**= 379

Clinical: Droperidol is a powerful tranquilizer. It is sometimes used as preanesthetic medication in labor and delivery because of fewer respiratory effects in neonates. It apparently crosses the placenta only very slowly. There are no data available on secretion into breastmilk. Due to the potent sedative properties of this medication, caution is urged.

DROSPERINONE AND ETHINYL ESTRADIOL; *Gianvi, Yasmin*	L3
Uses: Contraceptive	X
AAP: Not reviewed	

T½= 30.8, n/a; **RID**= ; **Oral** = 76%,40%; **MW**= 366.5(drospirenone), 296.4 (ethinyl estrodiol)

Clinical: Small amounts of oral contraceptive steroids have been identified in the milk of nursing mothers, and a few adverse effects on the child have been reported, including jaundice and breast enlargement. In addition, oral contraceptives given in the postpartum period may interfere with lactation by decreasing the quantity and quality of breast milk. If possible, the nursing mother should be advised not to use oral contraceptives but to use other forms of contraception until she has completely weaned her child.

DROTRECOGIN ALFA; *Xigris*	**L3**
Uses: Activated Protein C	**C**
AAP: Not reviewed	

T½= 1.6; **RID**= ; **Oral** = Nil; **MW**= 55,000

Clinical: No data are available on transfer to milk, but large molecular weight suggests it will be low. Unlikely to ever enter milk, or be orally bioavailable if it did.

DULOXETINE; *Cymbalta, Ariclaim, Duceten, Xeristar, Yentreve*	**L3**
Uses: Antidepressant	**C**
AAP: Not reviewed	

T½= 12 hours; **RID**= 0.1%; **Oral** = >70%; **MW**= 333

Clinical: Duloxetine is a selective serotonin and norepinephrine reuptake inhibitor (SNRI) similar in function to venlafaxine. It is indicated for major depressive disorders, and for diabetic peripheral neuropathic pain. New data suggest that the milk/plasma ratio is low (0.26%), and the RID (0.14%) is low as well. Daily dose is estimated to be 7 ug/day. This is too low to have clinical effects on an infant.

DYPHYLLINE; *Dilor, Lufyllin, Dyphylline, Broncho-Grippol*	**L3**
Uses: Anti-asthmatic drug	**C**
AAP: Maternal medication usually compatible with breastfeeding	

T½= 3-12.8 hours; **RID**= 42.3%; **Oral** = Complete; **MW**= 254

Clinical: Dyphylline is a methylxanthine, bronchodilator similar to theophylline. It is apparently secreted into milk in small quantities. No reported untoward effects. Observe infant for irritability, insomnia, and elevated heart rate.

ECHINACEA; *Echinacea angustifolia, Echinacea purpurea, American Cone Flower, Black Eyed Susan, Snakeroot*	L3
Uses: Herbal immunostimulant	
AAP: Not reviewed	
T½= ; RID= ; Oral = ; MW=	

Clinical: Echinacea is a popular herbal remedy in the central US and has been traditionally used topically to stimulate wound healing and internally to stimulate the immune system. The plant contains a complex mixture of compounds and, thus far, no single component appears responsible for its immunostimulant properties. No data are available on its transfer into human milk or its effect on lactation. It should not be used for more than 8 weeks.

ECONAZOLE; *Spectazole*	L3
Uses: Antifungal	C
AAP: Not reviewed	
T½= ; RID= ; Oral = ; MW= 381.7	

Clinical: Econazole Nitrate Cream, 1% is indicated for topical application in the treatment of tinea pedis, tinea cruris, and tinea corporis. It is not known whether econazole nitrate is excreted in human milk. Topically it is probably safe to use in a breastfeeding mother.

ECULIZUMAB; *Soliris*	L3
Uses: Monoclonal Antibody	C
AAP: Not reviewed	
T½= 272 hours; RID= ; Oral = Nil; MW= Large	

Clinical: Large antibody. Probably unable to penetrate milk compartment after first week. Levels in milk are probably undetectable. However, no data are yet available. It is extremely unlikely that this antibody would be transported into human milk, and due to its size, it would be largely unable to penetrate the milk compartment after the first week postpartum. Oral bioavailability would be nil.

EDROPHONIUM; *Enlon, Reversol, Tensilon*	**L3**
Uses: Cholinergic Agonist	**C**

AAP: Not reviewed

T½= 1.2-2.4 hours; **RID=** ; **Oral** = Nil; **MW=** 166

Clinical: Edrophonium is a rapid acetylcholinerase inhibitor. It also lasts briefly, only 10 minutes due to rapid redistribution out of the plasma. It is also a quarternary ammonium compound which means it would be unlikely to ever enter milk, or be orally absorbed.

EFALIZUMAB; *Raptiva*	**L3**
Uses: Monoclonal antibody	**C**

AAP: Not reviewed

T½= ; **RID=** ; **Oral** = Nil; **MW=** 150,000

Clinical: Efalizumab is an immunosuppressant used to treat moderate to severe plaque psoriasis. No data are available on the transfer of efalizumab into human milk. Because this antibody is quite large (150 kilodaltons), its size alone would prohibit its transfer into human milk in clinically relevant amounts.

EFAVIRENZ; *Sustiva, Atripla*	**L4**
Uses: Antiretroviral agent used in HIV infections.	**D**

AAP: Not reviewed

T½= not reported in humans; in monkeys = 42 %; **RID=** ; **Oral** = ; **MW=** 315.68

Clinical: There are no adequate and well-controlled studies in breastfeeding women. One study found that infant plasma concentrations were 13 % of the maternal plasma concentration in those who are breastfeeding. Breastfeeding is not recommended in mothers who have HIV.

EFLORNITHINE HYDROCHLORIDE; *Vaniqa*	**L3**
Uses: Hair growth retardant	**C**

AAP: Not reviewed

T½= 8 hours; **RID=** ; **Oral** = ; **MW=** 218

Clinical: Minimal transcutaneous absorption. Plasma levels are extraordinarily low. Levels in milk are likely low. A risk-benefit assessment of this product does not necessarily suggest the benefits are worth the risk for a breastfed infant, even if the risks are quite low.

ELETRIPTAN; *Relpax*	L2
Uses: Anti-migraine	C
AAP: Not reviewed	

T½= 4 hours; **RID**= 0.02%; **Oral** = 50%; **MW**= 463

Clinical: Eletriptan is a selective 5-hyroxytryptamine receptor agonists pecifically use to treat migraine attacks. The bioavailability of eletriptan is greater than sumatriptan(Imitrex) and is faster acting. The manufacturer reports that 0.02% of the administered dose is present in milk. It is not likely the clinical dose delivered above would harm a breastfed infant.

EMTRICITABINE + TENOFOVIR DISOPROXIL FUMARATE; *Truvada*	L4
Uses: Antiretroviral agent, reverse transcriptase inhibitor	B
AAP: Not reviewed	

T½= 10 hours; 17 hours; **RID**= ; **Oral** = 92%; 25%; **MW**= 247 for emtricitabine, 636 for tenofovir

Clinical: Used to treat HIV infections. It is not known whether tenofovir is excreted in human milk. It is not known whether emtricitabine is excreted in human milk. Because of both the potential for HIV-1 transmission and the potential for serious adverse reactions in nursing infants, mothers should be instructed not to breast-feed.

EMTRICITABINE; *Emtriva*	L4
Uses: Antiretroviral agent, reverse transcriptase inhibitor	B
AAP: Not reviewed	

T½= 10 hours; **RID**= ; **Oral** = Capsule: 93%; Solution: 75%; **MW**= 247

Clinical: It is not known whether emtricitabine is excreted in human milk. Because of both the potential for HIV-1 transmission and the potential for serious adverse reactions in nursing infants, mothers should be instructed not to breast-feed.

ENALAPRIL MALEATE; *Vasotec*	L2
Uses: Antihypertensive, ACE inhibitor	C

AAP: Maternal medication usually compatible with breastfeeding

T½= 35 hours (metabolite); **RID**= 0.2%; **Oral** = 60%; **MW**= 492

Clinical: Enalapril maleate is an ACE inhibitor used as an antihypertensive. Levels in milk are very low. Some caution is recommended in using ACE inhibitors in mothers with premature infants due to possible renal toxicity.

ENCAINIDE; *Enkaid*	L3
Uses: Antiarrhythmic agent	B

AAP: Not reviewed

T½= 2-36 hours; **RID**= 2.1%; **Oral** = Variable; **MW**= 352

Clinical: Encainide is a local anesthetic-type antiarrhythmic agent. It was voluntarily removed from the market in 1999 but is available on a limited basis for certain patients with life-threatening arrhythmias. Encainide and its 3 active metabolites are excreted into human milk although levels are moderately low.

ENOXACIN; *Penetrex*	L3
Uses: Antibiotic	C

AAP: Not reviewed

T½= 3-6 hours; **RID**= ; **Oral** = 90%; **MW**=

Clinical: Enoxacin is a typical fluoroquinolone antibiotic similar to ciprofloxacin, norfloxacin, and others. No data are available on the transfer of enoxacin into human milk. See ofloxacin and norfloxacin as alternatives.

ENOXAPARIN; *Lovenox, Low Molecular Weight Heparin*	L3
Uses: Anticoagulant	B

AAP: Not reviewed

T½= 4.5 hours; **RID**= ; **Oral** = None; **MW**= 8000

Clinical: Enoxaparin has a relatively large molecular weight (8000 daltons), which limits transfer into human milk. Also, enoxaparin is not absorbed well orally. Thus, the effect on the breastfed infant is minimal and probably safe. A similar compound, dalteparin, has been studied and milk levels are extremely low as well. See dalteparin.

EPHEDRINE; *Vatronol Nose Drops, Amsec*	L4
Uses: Adrenergic stimulant, anti-asthmatic	C
AAP: Not reviewed	

T½= 3-5 hours; **RID**= ; **Oral** = 85%; **MW**= 165

Clinical: Ephedrine is a mild stimulant that belongs to the adrenergic family and functions similar to the amphetamines. Small amounts of d-isoephedrine, a close congener of ephedrine, is believed to be secreted into milk although no data is available on ephedrine itself. This product is commonly used to support blood pressure of parturients during delivery. On an acute basis, it is not likely to harm a breastfeeding infant. However, it should not be used regularly by breastfeeding mothers.

EPINEPHRINE; *Adrenalin, Sus-Phren, Medihaler, Primatene, Adrenalin, Bronkaid, Epi-pen*	L1
Uses: Stimulant	C
AAP: Not reviewed	

T½= 1 hour (inhalation); **RID**= ; **Oral** = Poor; **MW**= 183

Clinical: Epinephrine is a powerful adrenergic stimulant. Although likely to be secreted in milk, it is rapidly destroyed in the GI tract. It is unlikely that any would be absorbed by the infant unless in the early neonatal period or premature.

EPLERENONE; *Inspra*	L3
Uses: Aldosterone receptor antagonist	B
AAP: Not reviewed	

T½= ; **RID**= ; **Oral** = 69%; **MW**= 414

Clinical: No data are available. Some caution is recommended.

EPOETIN ALFA; *Epogen* °	L3
Uses: Stimulates red blood cell production	C

AAP: Not reviewed

T½= 4-13 hours; **RID=** ; **Oral** = Nil; **MW=** 30,400

Clinical: Epoetin alfa is a glycoprotein which stimulates red blood cell production. It has a molecular weight of 30,400 daltons, thus it likely transfers into milk poorly. Further, due to its protein nature, it would not likely be absorbed orally to any degree by the infant.

EPOPROSTENOL; *Flolan*	**L3**
Uses: Vasodilator, platelet function inhibitor	**B**

AAP: Not reviewed

T½= 6 minutes; **RID=** ; **Oral** = Nil; **MW=** 374

Clinical: Epoprostenol is a naturally occurring prostaglandin that is commonly used to treat primary pulmonary hypertension. It is rapidly metabolized and has a half-life of only 3-5 minutes. With the extraordinarily short half-life of this product, it is unlikely any would penetrate into milk, be retained for very long, or be stable in the infant's gut. Oral absorption by the infant is unlikely.

EPROSARTAN; *Teveten*	**L3**
Uses: Antihypertensive, angiotensin receptor blocker	**C**

AAP: Not reviewed

T½= 20 hours; **RID=** ; **Oral** = 13%; **MW=** 520

Clinical: Eprosartan is a angiotensin receptor blocker used in hypertension. No data are available on its use in breastfeeding mothers. Its use in mothers breastfeeding premature infants, or even infants less than 4 months should be avoided due to possible renal toxicity.

EPSTEIN-BARR VIRUS; *Mononucleosis, EBV*	**L3**
Uses: Herpesvirus infection (EBV)	

AAP: Not reviewed

T½= ; **RID=** ; **Oral** = ; **MW=**

Clinical: The Epstein-Barr virus (EBV) is one of the causes of infectious mononucleosis. EBV belongs to the herpesvirus family. Symptoms include fever, exudative pharyngitis, lymphadenopathy, hepatosplenomegaly, and atypical lymphocytosis. Close personal contact is generally required for transmission and it is not known if EBV is secreted into human milk, although it is likely. Studies by Kusuhara indicate that the seroprevalence of EBV at 12-23 months was the same in bottle-fed and in breastfed infants. This data suggests that breastmilk is not a significant source of early EBV infections.

EPTIFIBATIDE; *Integrilin*	L3
Uses: Antiplatelet agent	B
AAP: Not reviewed	

T½= 2.5 hours; **RID**= ; **Oral** = Nil; **MW**= 831

Clinical: Small peptide, but still too large to really enter milk in clinically relevant amounts. Due to peptide structure, it is unlikely to be orally bioavailable in an infant.

ERGONOVINE MALEATE; *Ergotrate*	L3
Uses: Postpartum uterine bleeding	X
AAP: Not reviewed	

T½= 0.5-2 hours; **RID**= 1.9%; **Oral** = >60%; **MW**= 441

Clinical: Ergonovine and its close congener, methylergonovine maleate, directly stimulate uterine and vascula smooth muscle contractions. They are primarily used to prevent/treat postpartum hemorrhage. Levels in mik are low. However, it may reduce prolactin levels and milk production. The prolonged use of ergot alkaloids should be avoided and can lead to severe gangrenous manifestations.

ERGOTAMINE TARTRATE; *Wigraine, Cafergot, Ergostat, Ergomar, DHE-45, Gynergen*	L4
Uses: Anti-migraine, inhibits prolactin	X
AAP: Drugs associated with significant side effects and should be given with caution	

T½= 21 hours (terminal); **RID**= ; **Oral** = <5%; **MW**= 581

Clinical: Ergotamine is a potent vasoconstrictor generally used in acute phases of migraine headache. Excessive dosing and prolonged administration may inhibit prolactin secretion and hence lactation. Use during lactation should be strongly discouraged.

ERTAPENEM; *Invanz*	L2
Uses: Carbapenem antibiotic	B
AAP: Not reviewed	

T½= 4 hours; **RID**= 0.1% - 0.4%; **Oral** = Poor; **MW**= 497

Clinical: Levels in milk are reportedly very low. Most all the penicillins and the carbapenems are safe to use in breastfeeding mothers. Observe for changes in gut flora, diarrhea, etc.

ERYTHROMYCIN; *E-Mycin, Ery-Tab, Eryc, Ilosone, Eryc, Erythromide, Novo-Rythro, PCE, Ilotyc*	L2
Uses: Macrolide antibiotic	B
AAP: Maternal medication usually compatible with breastfeeding	

T½= 1.5-2 hours; **RID**= 1.4% - 1.7%; **Oral** = Variable; **MW**= 734

Clinical: Erythromycin transfer into milk is negligible, but it is apparently enough to increase the risk of pyloric stenosis in infants less than 13 days old. While this is probably somewhat remote, azithromycin is a nice substitute. A recent and large study now suggests a strong positive correlation between the use of erythromycin in breastfeeding mothers and infantile pyloric stenosis in newborns.

ESCITALOPRAM; *Lexapro*	L2
Uses: Antidepressant	C
AAP: Not reviewed	

T½= 27-32 hours; **RID**= 5.2% - 8%; **Oral** = 80%; **MW**= 414

Clinical: Recent and good data now show that levels in milk are low, and that plasma levels of escitalopram are low to undetectable in most infants. While the numbers are still low, it would appear this medication is probably safe to use in breastfeeding mothers.

ESMOLOL; *Brevibloc*	L3
Uses: Beta blocker antiarrhythmic	C

AAP:　Not reviewed

T½= 9 minutes;　**RID**= ;　**Oral** = Poor;　**MW**= 295

Clinical: Esmolol is an ultra short-acting beta blocker agent with low lipid solubility. It is only used IV and has an extremely short half-life. It is almost completely hydrolyzed in 30 minutes. No data on breastmilk levels are available.

ESOMEPRAZOLE; *Nexium*	L2
Uses:　Reduces gastric acid secretion	C

AAP:　Not reviewed

T½= 1-1.5 hours;　**RID**= ;　**Oral** = 90%;　**MW**= 345.4

Clinical: Esomeprazole poses little risk to a breastfeeding infant. Levels in milk are low, and it is unstable in the stomach at low pH.

ESTAZOLAM; *Prosom*	L3
Uses:　Benzodiazepine sedative	X

AAP:　Not reviewed

T½= 10-24 hours;　**RID**= ;　**Oral** = Complete;　**MW**= 295

Clinical: Estazolam is a benzodiazepine sedative hypnotic that belongs to the Valium family. No data are available on human milk levels. It is likely that some is secreted into human milk as well. The short-term risk to a breastfed infant is probably low.

ESTRIOL; *Ovestin Oestriol*	L3
Uses:　Estrogen	X

AAP:　Not reviewed

T½= ;　**RID**= ;　**Oral** = vaginal greater than oral;　**MW**=

Clinical: Estriol is a naturally secreted estrogen, typically during pregnancy in large quantities. Estriol usage is not indicated during lactation. Vaginal administration has systemic bioavailability similar to or greater than oral administration; estriol vaginal delivery may interfere with milk production as well.

ESTROGEN-ESTRADIOL; *Estratab, Premarin, Menext, Elestrin, Estrace, Estraderm, Delestrogen, Estinyl, Estring*	L3
Uses:　Estrogen hormone	X

AAP: Maternal medication usually compatible with breastfeeding

T½= 60 minutes; **RID=** ; **Oral** = Complete, vaginal 77%; **MW=** 272

Clinical: Estrogen transfer into human milk is low and clinical effects in the infant are unlikely. However, estrogens may suppress milk synthesis and mothers should be advise to avoid estrogen-containing products of any kind during lactation.

ESZOPICLONE; *Lunesta*	L3
Uses: Hypnotic, sedative	C
AAP: Not reviewed	

T½= 6 hours; **RID=** ; **Oral** = >75%; **MW=** 388

Clinical: Use of sedatives in breastfeeding mothers is of some concern, particularly those with premature or young neonates, and those with weak infants. This drug should be avoided in mothers with infants subject to apnea. Infant withdrawal has been reported following long-term use of benzodiazepines and could presumably occur with this agent as well. In mothers with healthy, older infants (> 2 months), there is probably little risk. Observe for poor feeding, apnea, and sedation.

ETANERCEPT; *Enbrel*	L3
Uses: Anti-arthritic	B
AAP: Not reviewed	

T½= 115 hours; **RID=** ; **Oral** = Nil; **MW=** 150000

Clinical: Etanercept is a large molecular IgG protein. While IgA is transported into milk, only small amounts of human IgG are transported. The one study that was published showing small levels of etanercept in milk was flawed in that milk was used from a mother who was not breastfeeding, and had already gone through involution of the breast. However, incredibly small amounts may still be present in milk, but it is not likely to ever survive the GI tract of the infant once ingested.

ETHACRYNIC ACID; *Edecrin*	L3
Uses: Powerful loop diuretic	B
AAP: Not reviewed	

T½= 2-4 hours; **RID=** ; **Oral** = 100%; **MW=** 303

Clinical: Ethacrynic acid is a potent, short-acting loop diuretic similar to Lasix. No data on transfer into human milk are available.

ETHAMBUTOL; *Ethambutol, Myambutol, Etibi*	L2
Uses: Antitubercular drug	B

AAP: Maternal medication usually compatible with breastfeeding

T½= 3.1 hours; **RID**= 1.5%; **Oral** = 80%; **MW**= 204

Clinical: Ethambutol is an antimicrobial used for tuberculosis. Small amounts are secreted in milk although no studies are available which clearly document levels.

ETHANOL; *Alcohol*	L3
Uses: Depressant	D

AAP: Maternal medication usually compatible with breastfeeding

T½= 0.24 hours; **RID**= 16%; **Oral** = 100%; **MW**= 46

Clinical: Heavy users should be advised not to breastfeed. Occasional users should use in limited quantities. A good rule is to wait 2 hours for every drink before returning to breastfeeding unless large quantities have been consumed, then the mother should wait longer.

ETHOSUXIMIDE; *Zarontin*	L4
Uses: Anticonvulsant used in epilepsy	C

AAP: Maternal medication usually compatible with breastfeeding

T½= 30-60 hours; **RID**= 31.5%; **Oral** = Complete; **MW**= 141

Clinical: A significant amount of ethosuximide is transferred into human milk. Monitoring for sedation, poor suckling, and hyperexcitability in the breastfed infant is advised. Ethosuximide is not the preferred choice as an antiepileptic, almost any other antiepileptic is a better choice (carbamazepine, gabapentin). Caution is recommended.

ETHOTOIN; *Peganone*	L3
Uses: Anticonvulsant	D

AAP: Not reviewed

T½= 3-9 hours; **RID**= ; **Oral** = Complete; **MW**= 204

Clinical: Ethotoin is a typical phenytoin-like anticonvulsant. Although no data is available on concentrations in breastmilk, its similarity to phenytoin would suggest that some is secreted via breastmilk. No data are available in the literature. See phenytoin.

ETIDRONATE; *Didronel*	L3
Uses: Slows bone turnover	C
AAP: Not reviewed	

T½= 6 hours (plasma); **RID**= ; **Oral** = 1-2.5%; **MW**= 206

Clinical: Etidronate is a bisphosphonate that slows the dissolution of hydroxyapatite crystals in the bone, thus reducing bone calcium loss in certain syndromes such as Paget's syndrome. Etidronate is poorly absorbed orally (1%) and must be administered in between meals on an empty stomach. Its penetration into milk is possible due to its small molecular weight, but it has not yet been reported. However, due to the presence of fat and calcium in milk, its oral bioavailability in infants would be exceedingly low.

ETODOLAC; *Etodolac, Lodine, Ultradol*	L3
Uses: Non-steroidal analgesic, antipyretic	C
AAP: Not reviewed	

T½= 7.3 hours; **RID**= ; **Oral** = 80-100%; **MW**= 287

Clinical: Etodolac is a typical nonsteroidal anti-inflammatory agent (NSAID) with analgesic, antipyretic, and anti-inflammatory properties. Thus far no data are available regarding its secretion into human breastmilk. Shorter half-life varieties are preferred such as ibuprofen and acetaminophen

---

ETONOGESTREL + ETHINYL ESTRADIOL; *NuvaRing*	L3
Uses: Slow release vaginal ring contraceptive	X
AAP: Not reviewed	

T½= 29.3 hours; **RID**= ; **Oral** = ; **MW**= 324

Clinical: NuvaRing is a slow release vaginal ring which releases on average 0.120 mg/day of etonogestrel and 0.015 mg/day of ethinyl estradiol over a 3 week period of use. Etonogestrel is the biologically active metabolite of desogestrel and has both high progestational activity with low intrinsic androgenicity. Small amounts of estrogens and progestins are known to pass into milk, but long-term follow-up of children whose mothers used combination hormonal contraceptives while breastfeeding has shown no deleterious effects on infants. Estrogen-containing contraceptives may interfere with milk production by decreasing the quantity and quality of milk production.

ETONOGESTREL IMPLANT; *Implanon*	L2
Uses: Implantable progestin contraceptive	X

AAP: Not reviewed

T½= 29.3 hours; **RID=** ; **Oral =** ; **MW=** 324

Clinical: Pure progestin. Probably a good choice for breastfeeding mothers. Transfer into milk is minimal and long-term complications in infant are unreported. Of the contraceptives, progestin-only contraceptives are generally preferred as they produce fewer changes in milk production compared to estrogen-containing products. This product is probably quite safe for use in breastfeeding mothers, although all mothers should be counseled to observe for changes in milk production.

ETRAVIRINE; *Intelence*	L4
Uses: Antiretroviral agent used in HIV infections. Antiretroviral drug	B

AAP: Not reviewed

T½= ; **RID=** ; **Oral =** ; **MW=**

Clinical: There are no adequate and well-controlled studies or case reports in breastfeeding women. Breastfeeding is not recommended in mothers who have HIV.

ETRETINATE; *Tegison*	L5
Uses: Antipsoriatic	X

AAP: Not reviewed

T½= 120 days (terminal); **RID=** ; **Oral =** Complete; **MW=** 354

Clinical: This product remains in adipose tissue for long periods and could over time transfer into human milk and produce clinical ranges in the infant. Great caution is recommended with breastfeeding following the use of this product.

EXENATIDE; *Byetta*	L3
Uses: Improves glycemic control in diabetics	C
AAP: Not reviewed	

T½= 2.4 hours; **RID**= ; **Oral** = Nil; **MW**= 4186

Clinical: The plasma levels of this product are extraordinarily low (peak is only 211 pg/mL), and I would imagine the transfer into human milk is much lower. It would be unlikely that this product would enter milk in clinically relevant amounts, nor would it be orally bioavailable in infants. But as yet, we have no data in breastfeeding mothers and caution is recommended if this product is used. Be slightly more cautious the first week postpartum before onset of mature milk.

EZETIMIBE; *Zetia*	L3
Uses: Anti-cholesterol agent	C
AAP: Not reviewed	

T½= 22 hours; **RID**= ; **Oral** = 35-60%; **MW**= 409

Clinical: Ezetimibe reduces blood cholesterol by inhibiting the absorption of cholesterol from the small intestine. No data are available on the transfer of this agent to milk. This is a very lipophilic agent, but has poor oral bioavailability. It is not clear at all if it would be safe for use in a breastfed infant who needs high levels of cholesterol. Some caution is recommended until data are available but it is unlikely to produce significant levels in milk.

FAMCICLOVIR; *Famvir*	L2
Uses: Antiviral for Herpes Zoster	B
AAP: Not reviewed	

T½= 2-3 hours; **RID**= ; **Oral** = 77%; **MW**=

Clinical: Famciclovir is probably safe to use during breastfeeding. We have no data on its transfer into human milk. Because famciclovir provides few advantages over acyclovir, at this point acyclovir would probably be preferred in a nursing mother although the side-effect profile is still minimal with this product.

FAMOTIDINE; *Pepcid, Axid-AR, Pepcid-AC, Apo-Famotidine, Novo-Famotidine*

L1

Uses: Reduces gastric acid secretion

B

AAP: Not reviewed

T½= 2.5-3.5 hours; **RID=** 1.9%; **Oral =** 50%; **MW=** 337

Clinical: Levels in milk are low. Famotidine is safe to use during breastfeeding and is the preferred choice in the Histamine-2 Antagonists drug class since lower levels of famotidine are found in breast milk.

FELBAMATE; *Felbatol*

L4

Uses: Anticonvulsant

C

AAP: Not reviewed

T½= 20-23 hours; **RID=** ; **Oral =** 90%; **MW=** 238

Clinical: Felbamate is an oral antiepileptic agent for partial seizures. Due to serious side effects, the FDA recommends that felbamate be given only to patients with serious seizures refractory to all other medications. No data are available on human milk. Due to the incidence of severe side effects, extreme caution is recommended with this medication in breastfeeding mothers.

FELODIPINE; *PlendilL, Plendil, Renedil*

L3

Uses: Calcium channel blocker, antihypertensive

C

AAP: Not reviewed

T½= 11-16 hours; **RID=** ; **Oral =** 20%; **MW=** 384

Clinical: Felodipine is a calcium channel antagonist structurally related to nifedipine. Because we have numerous studies on others in this family, it is advisable to use nifedipine or others that have breastfeeding studies available.

FENDOLOPAM; *Corlopam*

L3

Uses: Dopamine agonist

B

AAP: Not reviewed

T½= 5 minutes; **RID=** ; **Oral =** ; **MW=** 305

Clinical: Brief half-life. Unlikely to produce clinical levels in milk. Oral bioavailability is unknown. Dopamine agonists are known to suppress prolactin release, so some concern exists for the use of this product in breastfeeding mothers.

FENNEL; *Sweet Fennel, Bitter fennel, Carosella, Florence fennel, Finocchio, Garden fennel, Wild fennel*	L4

Uses: Estrogenic

AAP: Not reviewed

$T\frac{1}{2}$= ; **RID**= ; **Oral** = ; **MW**=

Clinical: No data concerning its use in breastfeeding mothers are available. It does however have some estrogenic properties which could suppress milk production. Caution is recommended. Because estrogens are known to suppress breastmilk production, its use in lactating women is questionable.

FENOFIBRATE; *Tricor*	L3
	C

Uses: Cholesterol lower agent

AAP: Not reviewed

$T\frac{1}{2}$= 20 hours; **RID**= ; **Oral** = 85%; **MW**= 361

Clinical: No data are available on its transfer into human milk however agents that reduce plasma cholesterol are not usually considered suitable for use in breastfeeding mothers.

FENOPROFEN; *Nalfon*	L2
	C

Uses: NSAID, nonsteroidal analgesic

AAP: Not reviewed

$T\frac{1}{2}$= 2.5 hours; **RID**= ; **Oral** = 80%; **MW**= 242

Clinical: Fenoprofen is a typical nonsteroidal antiinflammatory and analgesic. Fenoprofen levels in milk are too low to be accurately detected. Fenoprofen was undetectable in cord blood, amniotic fluid, saliva, or washed red blood cells after multiple doses. Suitable alternatives include ibuprofen or ketorolac.

FENTANYL; *Sublimaze, Onsolis, Duragesic*	L2
	C

Uses: Opiate analgesic

AAP: Maternal medication usually compatible with breastfeeding

$T\frac{1}{2}$= 2-4 hours; **RID**= 2.9% - 5%; **Oral** = 25-75%; **MW**= 336

Clinical: Fentanyl is probably safe to use during breastfeeding since only low levels pass into milk. There have been no reports of adverse effects in the breastfed infant. If the infant has a history of apnea, caution is advised.

FENUGREEK	L3

Uses: Herbal spice

AAP: Not reviewed

T½= ; **RID=** ; **Oral =** ; **MW=**

Clinical: Fenugreek is reported to be a galactagogue, although the effectiveness is questionable and not confirmed in literature. There seems to be minimal risk during breastfeeding when used in low-moderate doses.

FEXOFENADINE; *Allegra*	L2

Uses: Antihistamine   C

AAP: Maternal medication usually compatible with breastfeeding

T½= 14.4 hours; **RID=** 0.5% - 0.7%; **Oral =** Complete; **MW=** 538

Clinical: Fexofenadine is ideal and safe to use in breastfeeding since it is non-sedating, and transfers minimally to the breast milk. Other suitable antihistamines are loratadine and cetirizine. There have been no adverse effects reported in the breastfed infant.

FILGRASTIM; *Neupogen*	L2

Uses: Synthetic hematopoietic agent   C

AAP: Not reviewed

T½= 3.5 hours; **RID=** ; **Oral =** None; **MW=** 18,800

Clinical: Filgrastim is a large molecular weight biosynthetic protein used to stimulate blood cell production. There are no data on its entry into human milk, but due to its large molecular weight (18,800 daltons) it is very unlikely any would enter milk. Following use, the plasma levels in most individuals is often undetectable or in the picogram range. Further, due to its protein structure, it would not likely be orally bioavailable to the infant.

FLAVOXATE; *Urispas*	L3

Uses: Urinary antispasmodic   B

AAP: Not reviewed

T½= <10 hours; **RID=** ; **Oral =** Complete; **MW=** 391

Clinical: Flavoxate is use as an antispasmodic to provide relief of painful urination, urgency, nocturia, urinary frequency, or incontinence. No data are available on its transfer into human milk.

FLECAINIDE ACETATE; *Tambocor*	L3
Uses: Antiarrhythmic agent	C

AAP: Maternal medication usually compatible with breastfeeding

T½= 7-22 hours; **RID**= 4.9% - 5.2%; **Oral** = 90%; **MW**= 414

Clinical: Flecainide is a potent antiarrhythmic used to suppress dangerous ventricular arrhythmias. Levels in milk are moderate to very low. Some caution is recommended.

FLOXACILLIN; *Flucil, Fluclox*	L1
Uses: Penicillin antibiotic	B

AAP: Not reviewed

T½= 1.5 hours; **RID**= ; **Oral** = 50%; **MW**= 454

Clinical: Floxacillin is safe to use during breastfeeding, and is commonly used to treat mastitis in breastfeeding mothers with no adverse effects. Changes in gut flora is possible. Observe for diarrhea in the breastfed infant.

FLUCONAZOLE; *Diflucan*	L2
Uses: Antifungal, particularly candida infections	C

AAP: Maternal medication usually compatible with breastfeeding

T½= 30 hours; **RID**= 16.4% - 21.5%; **Oral** = >90%; **MW**= 306

Clinical: Transfer into milk is moderate (16-21%). However, no untoward effects have been reported in breastfed infants. However, recent studies bring into question the actual presence of candida albicans in breast milk or the ductal system. Hence, the use of this product in treating breast candidiasis is in question. Probably safe in most instances.

FLUDEOXYGLUCOSE F 18; *Fludeoxyglucose F 18*	L3
Uses: PET Scanning pharmaceutical	C

AAP: Not reviewed

T½= 110 minutes; **RID**= ; **Oral** = Complete; **MW**=

Clinical: Fludeoxyglucose F 18 is a radioactive pharmaceutical. Levels in milk are quite high. The calculated maximum cumulative dose to the infant, 0.085 mSv with no interruption of breast-feeding, is well below the recommended limit of 1 mSv. Indeed, a higher radiation dose is received by the infant from close contact with the breast than from ingestion of radioactive milk. The authors suggest pumping of the milk and feeding in bottles by another individual to reduce direct exposure to radiation. The USPDI(1994) recommends interruption of breastfeeding for 12-24 hours. At 9 hours, 97% of the radioisotope would be decayed away. It is likely that after 12 hours, almost all radioisotope would be decayed to almost background levels. Recommend pumping and dumping of breastmilk after the procedure for at least 12 hours to avoid all radiation.

FLUDROCORTISONE; *Florinef, Myconef*	L3
Uses: Mineralocorticoid	C

AAP: Not reviewed

T½= 3.5 hours; **RID**= ; **Oral** = Complete; **MW**= 380

Clinical: Fludrocortisone is a very potent steroid. It is not known if fludrocortisone penetrates into milk but if it is similar to other corticosteroids, it is very unlikely the amounts in milk will be clinically relevant until extremely high doses are used, but caution is recommended.

FLUNARIZINE; *Sibelium, Novo-Flunarizine*	L4
Uses: Antihypertensive	C

AAP: Not reviewed

T½= 19 days; **RID**= ; **Oral** = Complete; **MW**= 404

Clinical: Flunarizine is a calcium channel blocker primarily indicated for use in migraine headache prophylaxis and peripheral vascular disease. It has a very long half-life. No data are available on the transfer of this product into human milk. However, due to its incredibly long half-life and high volume of distribution, it is possible that this product, over time, could build up and concentrate in a breastfed infant. Other calcium channel blockers may be preferred. Use with extreme caution.

FLUNISOLIDE; *Nasalide, Aerobid, Bronalide, Rhinalar, PMS-Flunisolide*	L3
Uses: Inhaled and intranasal steroid	C

AAP: Not reviewed

T½= 1.8 hours; **RID**= ; **Oral** = 21% (oral); **MW**= 435

Clinical: Flunisolide is a potent corticosteroid used in asthmatics. It is also available as Nasalide for intranasal use for allergic rhinitis. Generally, only small levels of flunisolide are absorbed systemically (about 40%) thereby reducing systemic effects and presumably breastmilk levels as well. Although no data on breastmilk levels are yet available, it is unlikely that the level secreted in milk is clinically relevant.

FLUNITRAZEPAM; *Rohypnol*	L3
Uses: Benzodiazepine sedative	D

AAP: Not reviewed

T½= 20-30 hours; **RID**= ; **Oral** = 80-90%; **MW**= 313

Clinical: Flunitrazepam is a prototypic benzodiazepine. Frequently called the "Date Rape Pill", it induces rapid sedation and significant amnesia, particularly when mixed with alcohol. Effects last about 8 hours. It is recommended for adult insomnia and for pediatric preanesthetic sedation.

FLUOCINOLONE + HYDROQUINONE + TRETINOIN; *Tri-Luma*	L3
Uses: Treatment of melasma of the face	C

AAP: Not reviewed

T½= ; **RID**= ; **Oral** = ; **MW**=

Clinical: See individual monographs. The transcutaneous absorption of this product is moderate to minimal depending on the individual agent. Expect milk levels to be low, although we do not as yet have data on levels in breast milk. We do not have specific data on this combination product, but levels of the individual products are not high and milk levels will be much lower. However, caution is still recommended and a risk: benefit analysis must justify its use in breastfeeding mothers.

FLUORESCEIN; *AK-Fluor, Fluorescite, Funduscein-10, Ophthifluor, Fluorescein sodium, Ful-Glo, Fluorets, Fluor-I-Strip*	L3
Uses: Diagnostic dye in angiography	X

AAP: Maternal medication usually compatible with breastfeeding

T½= 4.4 hours (metabolite); **RID=** 0.8%; **Oral =** 50%; **MW=** 376

Clinical: Sodium fluorescein is a yellow, water-soluble dye. A 2% fluorescein ophthalmic solution or an impregnated fluorescein strip is used topically to detect corneal abrasions, for fitting of hard contact lenses, and intravenously for fluorescein angiography. Levels in milk appear low, but fluorescein-induced phototoxicity remains a possibility in an infant fed breastmilk containing sodium fluorescein. One case of severe fluorescein phototoxicity has been reported in an infant receiving fluorescein intravenously. If the infant is not undergoing phototherapy, it would appear that there is little risk to a breastfeeding infant.

FLUORIDE; *Pediaflor, Flura, Fluor-A-Day, Fluotic*	L2
Uses: Hardening enamel of teeth	C

AAP: Reported as having no effect on breastfeeding

T½= 6 hours; **RID=** ; **Oral =** 90% (Na); **MW=** 19

Clinical: Fluoride is an essential element required for bone and teeth development. It is available as salts of sodium and stannic (tin). Excessive levels are known to stain teeth irreversibly. Maternal supplementation is unnecessary and not recommended in areas with high fluoride content (>0.7 ppm) in water. The American Academy of Pediatrics no longer recommends supplementing of breastfed infants with oral fluoride for the first 6 months of life. From 6 months to 3 years of age, supplement fluoride drops only if drinking water levels are less than 0.3 ppm. Bottled water may or may not contain fluoride.

FLUOROURACIL; *5FU, Adrucil, Efudex, Fluoroplex, Carac*	L5
Uses: Anticancer drug, actinic keratosis	D

AAP: Not reviewed

T½= 8-22 minutes; **RID=** ; **Oral =** 0-80%; **MW=** 130

Clinical: 5-Fluorouracil is a potent and dangerous antineoplastic agent. Antineoplastic activity is dependent on the intracellular activation of 5FU itself. Thus prolonged IV infusions are often used to enhance potentcy. It is well absorbed orally, but poorly absorbed transcutaneously. Milk levels have not yet been published. Breastfeeding is probably fine if exposure is due to topical application over small to moderate areas (not large areas). If used orally, or intravenously in significant doses, a suitable waiting period should be used to avoid exposure of the infant. Because it has only a 12 minute half-life, a few hours, or better, 24 hours would probably reduce any risk from this agent. The injection into the intraocular space would prolong the release of 5FU into the plasma. But the dose is so low, it is unlikely to cause significant exposure to a breastfeeding infant via breastmilk.

FLUOXETINE; *Prozac, Apo-Fluoxetine, Novo-Fluoxetine*	L2
Uses: Antidepressant	C

AAP: Drugs whose effect on nursing infants is unknown but may be of concern

T½= 2-3 days (fluoxetine); **RID**= 1.6% - 14.6%; **Oral** = 100%; **MW**= 309

Clinical: Fluoxetine, while perhaps not the best SSRI has been used in perhaps a million breastfeeding mothers over the last 2 decades. While there are some reports of complications, they are in general minimal and may actually be discontinuation syndrome rather than serotonin syndrome from the medication. While sertraline and escitalopram levels in milk are probably lower, fluoxetine is quite suitable for breastfeeding mothers and their infants. Remember, the risk of untreated depression is far higher than the risks of this medication.

FLUPHENAZINE; *Prolixin, Permitil, Apo-Fluphenazine, Modecate, Moditen*	L3
Uses: Psychotherapeutic agent	C

AAP: Not reviewed

T½= 10-20 hours; **RID**= ; **Oral** = Complete; **MW**= 438

Clinical: Fluphenazine is a phenothiazine tranquilizer and presently has the highest milligram potency of this family. Long half-life. No data are available on this medication in breastfeeding mothers. Caution.

FLURAZEPAM; *Dalmane, Apo-Flurazepam, Novo-Flupam*	L3
Uses: Sedative, hypnotic	X
AAP: Not reviewed	
T½= 47-100 hours; **RID=** ; **Oral** = Complete; **MW=** 388	
Clinical: Caution is advised when using flurazepam during breastfeeding. We have no data on its transfer into human milk. Observe for sedation in the breastfed infant. A suitable alternative is lorazepam.	

FLURBIPROFEN; *Ansaid, Froben, Ocufen*	L2
Uses: Analgesic	B
AAP: Not reviewed	
T½= 3.8-5.7 hours; **RID=** 0.7% - 1.4%; **Oral** = Complete; **MW=** 244	
Clinical: Flurbiprofen is a nonsteroidal analgesic similar in structure to ibuprofen but used both as an ophthalmic preparation (in eyes) and orally. Levels in milk are exceedingly low. Two studies suggest that the amount of flurbiprofen transferred in human milk would be clinically insignificant to the infant.	

FLUTICASONE AND SALMETEROL; *Advair*	L3
Uses: Anti-asthmatic	C
AAP: Not reviewed	
T½= ; **RID=** ; **Oral** = ; **MW=**	
Clinical: Fluticasone is probably quite safe. Limited oral bioavailability and high first-pass uptake would limit maternal plasma levels. This product is used in children all the time. It would not be contraindicated in a breastfeeding mother. Salmeterol levels are undetectable in the maternal plasma after inhaled administration. The combined use of salmeterol and fluticasone is probably compatible with breastfeeding.	

FLUTICASONE; *Flonase, Flovent, Cutivate, Veramyst*	L3
Uses: Intranasal, inhaled steroid	C
AAP: Not reviewed	
T½= 7.8 hours; **RID=** ; **Oral** = Oral (1%), Inhaled (18%); **MW=** 500	

Clinical: Probably quite safe. Limited oral bioavailability and high first-pass uptake would limit maternal plasma levels. This product is used in children all the time. It would not be contraindicated in a breastfeeding mother. With the above limited oral and systemic bioavailability, and rapid first-pass uptake by the liver, it is not likely that milk levels will be clinically relevant, even with rather high doses.

FLUVASTATIN; *Lescol, Lescol XL*	L3
Uses: Reduces blood cholesterol levels	X
AAP: Not reviewed	
T½= 1.2 hours; **RID**= ; **Oral** = 20-30%; **MW**=	

Clinical: Fluvastatin is an inhibitor of cholesterol synthesis. Use of statins at this time are not recommended in breastfeeding mothers, although they probably pose little risk.

FLUVOXAMINE; *Luvox, Apo-Fluvoxamine, Alti-Fluvoxamine*	L2
Uses: Antidepressant	C
AAP: Drugs whose effect on nursing infants is unknown but may be of concern	
T½= 15.6 hours; **RID**= 0.3% - 1.4%; **Oral** = 53%; **MW**= 318	

Clinical: Works like other SSRIs, by increasing synaptic serotonin levels in the brain. Reported levels in milk are low and in some studies is undetectable in the infant. In summary, the data from 8 cases suggests that only minuscule amounts of fluvoxamine are transferred to infants, that plasma levels in infants are too low to be detected, and no adverse effects have been noted.

FOLIC ACID; *Folacin, Wellcovorin, Apo-Folic, Folvite, Novo-Folacid*	L1
Uses: Vitamin B-9	A
AAP: Maternal medication usually compatible with breastfeeding	
T½= ; **RID**= ; **Oral** = 76-93%; **MW**= 441	

Clinical: Safe. Higher doses are recommended in young females consuming anticonvulsants.

FOLLICLE STIMULATING HORMONES; *Metrodin, Fertinex, FSH, Follistim, Follitropin Alpha, Follitropin Beta, Gonal-F, Fertinorm HP*	L3
Uses: FSH, follicle stimulating hormone	X

AAP: Not reviewed

T½= 3.9 and 70.4 hours; **RID=** ; **Oral** = None; **MW**= 34,000

Clinical: Follicle-stimulating hormone is a large molecular weight protein. Found in normal menstruating women, it is unlikley to enter milk due to its large molecular weight.

FONDAPARINUX SODIUM; *Arixtra*	L3
Uses: Factor Xa inhibitor	B

AAP: Not reviewed

T½= 17-21 hours; **RID=** ; **Oral** = Nil; **MW**= 1728

Clinical: Small pentasaccharide that would not be orally bioavailable, nor likely to enter the milk compartment. No data are available on the transmission of fondaparinux sodium to a nursing infant, but based on the kinetic profile it is highly unlikely that it would be passed to the infant.

FORMALDEHYDE; *Formaldehyde, Formalin, Methyl aldehyde*	L4
Uses: Preservative	X

AAP: Not reviewed

T½= ; **RID=** ; **Oral** = ; **MW**= 30

Clinical: Formaldehyde exposure in laboratory or embalming environments is strictly controlled by federal regulations to a permissible level of 2 ppm. Formaldehyde is rapidly destroyed by plasma and tissue enzymes and it is very unlikely that any would enter human milk following environmental exposures. However, acute intoxications following high oral or inhaled doses could lead to significant levels of maternal plasma formic acid which could enter milk. There are no data suggesting untoward side effects in nursing infants as a result of mild to minimal environmental exposure of the mother.

FORMOTEROL FUMARATE; *Foradil Aerolizer, Symbicort*	L3
Uses: Bronchodilator	C

AAP: Not reviewed

T½= 10 hours; **RID=** ; **Oral** = Good; **MW=** 840

Clinical: Formoterol is used for asthma and COPD. No data are available on its transfer into human milk, but the extremely low plasma levels would suggest that milk levels would be incredibly low, if even measurable. Studies of oral absorption in adults suggests that while absorption is good, plasma levels are still below detectable levels and may require large oral doses prior to attaining measurable plasma levels. It is not likely the amount present in human milk would be clinically relevant to a breastfed infant.

FOSCARNET SODIUM; *Foscavir*	L4
Uses: Antiviral for herpes, CMV infections	C

AAP: Not reviewed

T½= 3 hours; **RID=** ; **Oral** = 12-21%; **MW=** 192

Clinical: Foscarnet is an antiviral used to treat herpes simplex manifestations and cytomegalovirus retinal infections in patients with AIDS. Foscarnet is a potent and potentially dangerous drug including significant renal toxicity, seizures, and deposition in bone and teeth. Caution.

FOSFOMYCIN TROMETAMOL; *Monurol*	L3
Uses: Urinary antibiotic	B

AAP: Not reviewed

T½= 4-8 hours; **RID=** ; **Oral** = 34-58%; **MW=** 138

Clinical: Fosfomycin is a broad-spectrum antibiotic used primarily for uncomplicated urinary tract infections. It is believed safe for use in pregnancy and has been used in children less than 1 year of age. Fosfomycin secreted into human milk would likely be in the calcium form and is unlikely to be absorbed as secreted in human milk. It is not likely that the levels present in breastmilk would produce untoward effects in a breastfeeding infant.

FOSINOPRIL; *Monopril*	L3
Uses: Antihypertensive, ACE inhibitor	C

AAP: Not reviewed

T½= 11-35 hours; **RID=** ; **Oral** = 30-36%; **MW=** 564

Clinical: Fosinopril is a prodrug that is metabolized by the gut and liver to an ACE inhibitor used as an antihypertensive. The manufacturer reports that the ingestion of 20 mg daily for three days resulted in barely detectable levels in human milk, although no values are provided.

FOSPHENYTOIN; *Cerebyx*	L2
Uses: Anticonvulsant	D

AAP: Not reviewed

T½= 15 minutes; **RID**= ; **Oral** = ; **MW**= 406

Clinical: Fosphenytoin is rapidly metabolized to phenytoin. See phenytoin monograph for data and comments.

FROVATRIPTAN SUCCINATE; *Frova*	L3
Uses: Anti-migraine, 5-HT1B/1D receptor agonist	C

AAP: Not reviewed

T½= 26 hours; **RID**= ; **Oral** = 30%; **MW**= 379

Clinical: Frovatriptan is used to treat migraine headaches. No data on its transfer to milk are available. Some studies suggest sumatriptan may be more effective. Sumatriptan is recommended as we have good data suggesting milk levels of sumatriptan are low and its oral bioavailability is low.

FURAZOLIDONE; *Furoxone*	L2
Uses: Gastrointestinal antibiotic	C

AAP: Not reviewed

T½= ; **RID**= ; **Oral** = <5%; **MW**= 225

Clinical: Furazolidone belongs to the nitrofurantoin family of antibiotics (see nitrofurantoin). It is poorly absorbed (<5%) and is largely inactivated in the gut. Concentrations transferred to milk are unreported, but the total amounts would be exceedingly low due to the low maternal plasma levels attained by this product. Due to poor oral absorption, systemic absorption in a breastfeeding infant would likely be minimal. Caution should be observed in early postpartum newborns due to hyperbilirubinemia.

FUROSEMIDE; *Lasix, Apo-Furosemide, Novo-Semide*	L3
Uses: Loop diuretic	C

AAP: Not reviewed

T½= 92 minutes; **RID**= ; **Oral** = 60-70%; **MW**= 331

Clinical: Furosemide is commonly used in infants in high doses due to low oral bioavailability, thus transfer through breast milk poses minimal risk. There is a theoretical possibility of decreased milk production.

GABAPENTIN; *Neurontin*	**L2**
Uses: Anticonvulsant	**C**

AAP: Not reviewed

T½= 5-7 hours; **RID**= 6.6%; **Oral** = 50-60%; **MW**=

Clinical: Levels in infants are low. Milk levels are low. Probably of minimal risk after the first month or so postpartum. No complications in infants in two studies. Still some caution is recommended.

GADOPENTETATE DIMEGLUMINE; *Gadolinium, Magnevist*	**L2**
Uses: Contrast agent	**C**

AAP: Not reviewed

T½= ; **RID**= ; **Oral** = ; **MW**=

Clinical: Levels in milk are exceedingly low from two studies. The cumulative amount excreted from both breasts in 24 hours was only 0.023% of the administered dose. Oral absorption is minimal, only 0.8% of gadopentetate is absorbed. Probably safe. One pumping and discarding at 3 hours would eliminate most risk.

GADOVERSETAMIDE; *Optimark*	**L3**
Uses: Magnetic Resonance Imaging Agent	**C**

AAP: Not reviewed

T½= 104; **RID**= ; **Oral** = 100%; **MW**=

Clinical: Gadoversetamide is a paramagnetic agent used in MRI. It was excreted in the milk of lactatin rats receiving a single intravenous dose of 0.1 mmol/kg. Women should discontinue nursing and discard breast milk up to 72 hours after administration.

GALLIUM-67 CITRATE; *Gallium-67 Citrate*	L4
Uses: Radioactive isotope	X

AAP: Radioactive compound that requires temporary cessation of breastfeeding

T½= 78.3 hours; **RID=** ; **Oral** = ; **MW=**

Clinical: A significant risk is associated with the use of this product in breastfeeding mothers and their infants. Approximations suggest that breastfeeding should be interrupted for a minimum of 1 week following a dose of 0.2 mCi, 2 weeks for 1.3 mCi, or 1 month for 4 mCi. Up to 1 month of no breastfeeding is required after 4 mCi dose.

GAMMA HYDROXYBUTYRIC ACID; *GBH,* *Gamma-OH, Somsanit, Oxybutyrate, GHB, Liquid Ecstasy*	L5
Uses: Illicit sedative, hallucinogen, growth stimulant	X

AAP: Not reviewed

T½= 20-60 minutes; **RID=** ; **Oral** = Good; **MW=** 126

Clinical: This is a strong neuroleptic drug and its use should be avoided by all breastfeeding mothers. It has a rather brief half-life (20-60 minutes) and < 5% remains in the plasma compartment following 10 hours, and virtually none is detected in the urine after 12 hours. While these levels would depend on the dose, if the patient has returned to normal, milk levels after 12 hours would probably be low to undetectable. Although we do not have milk levels reported, but they would probably be significant during peak exposure. In patients that have dosed repeatedly for hours, a 24 hour pump and discard would be advisable. This product is strongly additive with alcohol as it is metabolized by alcohol dehydrogenase. This is a dangerous product that should never be used in breastfeeding mothers. Mothers exposed to this agent should pump and discard their milk for a minimum of 12-24 hours depending on the dose before returning the infant to the breast.

GANIRELIX ACETATE; *Antagon*	L3
Uses: Synthetic gonotrophic-releasing hormone antagonist	X

AAP: Not reviewed

T½= 16.2 hours; **RID=** ; **Oral** = Nil; **MW=** 1570

Clinical: No data are available on the transfer of this decapeptide into human milk but it is unlikely due to its peptide structure and its larger molecular weight. In addition, it is very unlikely this decapeptide would be stable in the infants' GI tract or orally bioavailable.

GARLIC; *Allium, Stinkin rose, Rustic treacle, Camphor of the poor*	**L3**
Uses: Herbal antioxidant	
AAP: Not reviewed	

T½= ; **RID=** ; **Oral** = ; **MW=**

Clinical: Garlic contains a number of sulfur-containing compounds that, when ground, are metabolized to allicin, which is responsible for the pungent odor of garlic and the pharmacologic effects attributed to garlic. Although garlic oil is commonly used, the safety for long term use is still unresolved. The extract has caused a reduction in liver and kidney protein in animal studies and a potential interaction with other anticoagulants (warfarin) should be expected. Transfer of the odorous components in human milk has been documented. Do not overdose.

GATIFLOXACIN OPHTHALMIC SOLUTION; *Tequin, Zymar, Zymaxid*	**L3**
Uses: Fluoroquinolone anti-injective antibiotic	C
AAP: Not reviewed	

T½= 7.1 hours; **RID=** ; **Oral** = 96%; **MW=** 402

Clinical: We have no data on the transfer of this fluoroquinolone into human milk. The only major complication is a change in GI flora. Following the use of the ophthalmic forms of gatifloxacin, levels are so low that they are undetectable by one manufacturer, and only barely detectable by group.

GEMFIBROZIL; *Lopid, Gemcor, Apo-Gemfibrozil*	**L3**
Uses: Antilipemic agent	C
AAP: Not reviewed	

T½= 1.5 hours; **RID=** ; **Oral** = 97%; **MW=** 250

Clinical: Gemfibrozil is a hypolipidemic agent primarily used to lower triglyceride levels. There are no data on its transfer into human milk. Reproductive studies in rodents at high doses have not revealed any evidence of harm to the fetus. But the risks of using lipid lowering drugs while pregnant, and probably while breastfeeding, may be higher than the overall risks of hyperlipidemia and, therefore, are not usually justified.

GEMIFLOXACIN MESYLATE; *Factive*	L3
Uses: Antibiotic	C
AAP: Not reviewed	
T½= 7 hours; **RID**= ; **Oral** = 71%; **MW**= 485	

Clinical: Has high Vd, therefore milk levels are probably low. Some caution is recommended due to overgrowth of C.difficle. Observe for bloody diarrhea and changes in gut flora. But this product is probably less risky than ciprofloxacin.

GENTAMICIN; *Garamycin, Alocomicin, Cidomycin, Garatec*	L2
Uses: Aminoglycoside antibiotic	C
AAP: Maternal medication usually compatible with breastfeeding	
T½= 2-3 hours; **RID**= 2.1%; **Oral** = <1%; **MW**=	

Clinical: Gentamicin is a narrow spectrum antibiotic generally used for gram negative infections. The oral absorption of gentamicin (<1%) is generally nil with the exception of premature neonates, where small amounts may be absorbed. Levels in milk are very low and would be clinically insignificant.

GENTIAN VIOLET; *Crystal Violet, Methylrosaniline chloride, Gentian Violet*	L3
Uses: Antifungal, antimicrobial	C
AAP: Not reviewed	
T½= ; **RID**= ; **Oral** = ; **MW**= 408	

Clinical: Messy although quite effective for treatment of oral thrush in infants. Do not use concentrations higher than 1-2% 2-3 times daily, and no longer than 3-5 days. This product is irratation to mucous membrane.

GINGER	L3
Uses: Herb	C

AAP: Not reviewed

T½= ; **RID**= ; **Oral** = ; **MW**=

Clinical: There are no adequate and well-controlled studies or case reports in breastfeeding women. Safe in both pregnancy and probably breastfeeding.

GINKGO BILOBA; *Ginkgo*	L3
Uses: Herbal antioxidant	

AAP: Not reviewed

T½= ; **RID**= ; **Oral** = ; **MW**=

Clinical: No data are available on the transfer of GBE into human milk. Thus far, with exception of the seeds, GBE appears relatively non-toxic.

GINSENG; *Panax*	L3
Uses: Herbal tonic	

AAP: Not reviewed

T½= ; **RID**= ; **Oral** = ; **MW**=

Clinical: No data are available concerning the transfer into human milk. It is recommended that it not be used for more than 6 weeks.

GLATIRAMER; *Copaxone*	L3
Uses: Relapsing multiple sclerosis	B

AAP: Not reviewed

T½= ; **RID**= ; **Oral** = Minimal; **MW**= 4700+

Clinical: There are no data available on transfer of glatiramer into milk, however it is highly unlikely due to its large molecular weight. It is probably okay to use during breastfeeding. We have had case reports of infants that itch and scratch their face when breastfeeding shortly after the mother takes glatiramer. Suggest pumping and discarding milk after glatiramer administration and then waiting an hour before breastfeeding. A suitable alternative is interferon beta-1a, which is an even larger drug.

GLIMEPIRIDE; *Amaryl*	L4
Uses: Lowers plasma glucose	C

AAP: Not reviewed

T½= 6-9 hours; **RID=** ; **Oral** = 100%; **MW=** 490

Clinical: Glimepiride is used to lower plasma glucose in patients with non-insulin dependent diabetes mellitus. No data are available on the transfer of this product into human milk. However, rodent studies demonstrated significant transfer and elevated plasma levels in pups. Caution is recommended if used in breastfeeding humans. Observe for hypoglycemia.

GLIPIZIDE; *Glucotrol XL, Glucotrol*	L3
Uses: Prolonged release hypoglycemic agent	C

AAP: Not reviewed

T½= 4-6 hours; **RID=** ; **Oral** = 80-100%; **MW=** 446

Clinical: The transfer of glipizide to milk is apparently quite low. Levels in one study were below limit of detection (< 0.08 ug/ml). No changes in the infants plasma glucose levels were noted.

GLUCOSAMINE; *Glucosamine*	L3
Uses: Antiarthritic	

AAP: Not reviewed

T½= 0.3 hours; **RID=** ; **Oral** = <26%; **MW=** 179

Clinical: Glucosamine is an endogenous which is a constituent of cartilage proteoglycans. Administered in large doses, most is sequestered in the liver with only minimal amounts reaching other tissues, thus oral bioavailability is low. Most of the oral dose is hepatically metabolized and subsequently incorporated into other plasma proteins. No data are available on transfer into human milk. Because glucosamine is primarily sequestered and metabolized in the liver, and because the plasma levels are almost undetectable, it is unlikely that much would enter human milk.

GLYBURIDE; *Micronase, Diabeta, Glynase, Glucovance,* *Diabeta, Euglucon, Gen-Glybe*	L2
Uses: Hypoglycemic, antidiabetic agent	B

AAP: Not reviewed

T½= 4-13.7 hours; **RID=** ; **Oral** = Complete; **MW=** 494

Clinical: The transfer of glyburide to milk is apparently quite low. Levels in one study were below limit of detection (0.005 ug/ml). No changes in the infants plasma glucose levels were noted.

GLYCOPYRROLATE; *Robinul*	L3
Uses: Anticholinergic	B

AAP: Not reviewed

T½= 1.7 hours; **RID=** ; **Oral** = 10-25%; **MW=** 398

Clinical: Glycopyrrolate is an anticholinergic used prior to surgery to dry secretions. After administration, its plasma half-life is exceedingly short (<5 min.) with most of the product being distribution out of the plasma compartment rapidly. No data are available on its transfer into human milk, but due to its short plasma half-life and its quaternary structure, it is very unlikely that significant quantities would penetrate milk. Further, along with the poor oral bioavailability of this product, it is very remote that glycopyrrolate would pose a significant risk to a breastfeeding infant.

GOLD COMPOUNDS; *Ridaura, Myochrysine, Solganal, Myochrysine*	L5
Uses: Antiarthritic	C

AAP: Maternal medication usually compatible with breastfeeding

T½= 3-26 days; **RID=** 0.6% - 2.8%; **Oral** = 20-25% (auranofin); **MW=**

Clinical: Studies thus far are highly variable from a low of perhaps 0.75% of the maternal dose, to as high as 10% of the maternal dose. However, the oral absorption of gold in a humans is likely low (<20%) due to high protein binding, etc. So in reality, the risk to the infant is probably somewhat low. But gold is stored in the body for long periods (months), and chronic exposure to low levels of gold could lead to increasing levels in breastfed infants. This product is probably a little too risky to use in breastfeeding mothers. Other alternatives should be explored.

GONADORELIN ACETATE; *Lutrepulse*	L3
Uses: Gonadotropin-releasing hormone	B

AAP: Not reviewed

T½= 2-4 minutes; **RID=** ; **Oral** = None; **MW=**

Clinical: Gonadorelin is a small decapeptide identical to the physiologic peptide secreted in the human. Gonadorelin has been detected in human breastmilk at concentrations of 0.1 to 3 nanograms/mL (adult dose= 20-100 micrograms) although its oral bioavailability in the infant would be minimal to none.

GOSERELIN ACETATE IMPLANT; *Zoladex*	L3
Uses: Inhibitor of luteinizing hormone	X

AAP: Not reviewed

T½= 2.3 hours; **RID**= ; **Oral** = Nil; **MW**= 1269

Clinical: Goserelin is a synthetic decapeptide analogue of luteinizing hormone. No data are available on its transfer into human milk but due to its structure and molecular weight it is very unlikely to enter milk, or to be orally bioavailable in the infant.

GRANISETRON; *Kytril*	L3
Uses: Antiemetic	B

AAP: Not reviewed

T½= 3-14 hours; **RID**= ; **Oral** = 60%; **MW**= 349

Clinical: Granisetron is an antinauseant and antiemetic agent commonly used with chemotherapy. No data are available on its transfer into human milk but its levels are likely to be low. Further, this family of products (see ondansetron) are not highly toxic and are commonly used in children (2 years). It is unlikely that this product will be overtly toxic to a breastfed infant.

GREPAFLOXACIN; *Raxar*	L4
Uses: Fluoroquinolone antibiotic	C

AAP: Not reviewed

T½= 15.7 hours; **RID**= ; **Oral** = 72%; **MW**= 422

Clinical: Grepafloxacin is a typical fluoroquinolones antibiotic similar to Ciprofloxacin. The manufacturer suggests that grepafloxacin is detectable in human milk after a 400 mg dose but does not provide the exact levels. Others in this family are preferred.

GRISEOFULVIN; *Fulvicin, Gris-PEG, Grisovin-FP*	L2
Uses: Antifungal	C

AAP: Not reviewed

T½= 9-24 hours; **RID=** ; **Oral** = Poor to 50%; **MW=** 353

Clinical: Griseofulvin is an older class antifungal. Much better safety profiles with the newer families of antifungals have reduced the use of griseofulvin. This is not an ideal agent in breastfeeding mothers.

GUAIFENESIN; *GG, Robitussin, Mucinex, Balminil, Resyl, Benylin-E*	**L2**
Uses: Expectorant, loosens respiratory tract secretions	C

AAP: Not reviewed

T½= <7 hours; **RID=** ; **Oral** = Complete; **MW=** 198

Clinical: Antihistamine, expectorant. No data are available on transfer into human breastmilk. In general, clinical studies documenting the efficacy of guaifenesin are lacking, and the usefulness of this product as an expectorant is highly questionable. But probably safe.

HAEMOPHILUS B CONJUGATE VACCINE; *HibTITER, Haemophilus B Vaccine, Hiberix, ProHIBiT, OmniHIB, Act-HIB*	**L3**
Uses: H. influenza vaccine	C

AAP: Not reviewed

T½= ; **RID=** ; **Oral** = ; **MW=**

Clinical: Hib Vaccine is a polysaccharide vaccine made from Haemophilus influenza bacteria. It is non-infective. It is currently recommended for initial immunizations in children at 2 months, and at 2 month intervals, for a total of 3 injections. Although there are no reasons for administering to adult mothers, it would not be contraindicated in breastfeeding mothers.

HALAZEPAM; *Paxipam*	**L3**
Uses: Benzodiazepine antianxiety drug	D

AAP: Not reviewed

T½= 14 hours; **RID=** ; **Oral** = Complete; **MW=** 353

Clinical: Halazepam is a sedative medication used to treat anxiety disorders. Halazepam is metabolized to desmethyldiazepam, which has an elimination half-life of 50-100 hours. Although no information is available on halazepam levels in human milk, it should be similar to diazepam. See diazepam.

HALOPERIDOL; *Haldol, Apo-Haloperidol, Novo-Peridol, Peridol*	L2
Uses: Antipsychotic	C

AAP: Drugs whose effect on nursing infants is unknown but may be of concern

T½= 12-38 hours; **RID=** 2.1% - 12%; **Oral** = 60%; **MW=** 376

Clinical: Haloperidol is a potent antipsychotic agent that as a side effect may increase prolactin levels in some patients. Levels in milk are significant. Some caution is recommended in breastfeeding mothers.

HALOTHANE; *Fluothane*	L2
Uses: Anesthetic gas	C

AAP: Maternal medication usually compatible with breastfeeding

T½= ; **RID=** ; **Oral** = ; **MW=** 197

Clinical: Halothane is an anesthetic gas similar to enflurane, methoxyflurane, and isoflurane. Approximately 60-80% is rapidly eliminated by exhalation the first 24 hours. The authors assessed the exposure to the infant as negligible. Pumping and dumping milk the first 24 hours postoperatively is generally recommended but is probably unnecessary.

HCTZ + TRIAMTERENE; *Maxzide, Dyazide, Novo-Triamzide*	L3
Uses: Diuretic	C

AAP: Not reviewed

T½= 1.5-2.5 hours; **RID=** 0.2%; **Oral** = 30-70%; **MW=** 253

Clinical: See hydrochlorthiazide. Triamterene is a potassium sparing diuretic. It is secreted in small amounts in cow's milk but no human data are available. Levels in human milk are unlikely to be clinically relevant.

HEMIN; *Panhematin*	L3
Uses: Blood modifier	C

AAP: Not reviewed

T½= ; **RID=** ; **Oral** = Nil; **MW=** 616

Clinical: No data are available on the levels in breast milk. However, this is a large molecular weight protein that is unlikely to enter the milk compartment, nor be orally bioavailable to an infant.

HEPARIN; *Heparin, Hepalean*	L1
Uses: Anticoagulant	C

AAP: Not reviewed

T½= 1-2 hours; **RID=** ; **Oral** = None; **MW=** 12-15,000

Clinical: Heparin is safe to use during breastfeeding. It is very unlikely that heparin transfers into milk due to its large molecular structure. No adverse effects are expected in breastfed infants. Any present in milk would be rapidly destroyed in the gastric contents of the infant.

HEPATITIS A INFECTION	L3
Uses: Viral infection	

AAP: Not reviewed

T½= ; **RID=** ; **Oral** = ; **MW=**

Clinical: Hepatitis A is an acute viral infection characterized by jaundice, fever, anorexia, and malaise. In infants, the syndrome is either asymptomatic or causes only mild nonspecific symptoms. A majority of the population is immune to Hepatitis A due to prior exposure. Fulminant hepatitis A infection is rare in children and a carrier state is unknown. It is unlikely to bother a breastfeeding infant.

HEPATITIS B IMMUNE GLOBULIN; *H-BIG, HEP-B-Gammagee, Hyperhep*	L2
Uses: Anti-Hepatitis B Immune globulins	C

AAP: Not reviewed

T½= ; **RID=** ; **Oral** = None; **MW=**

Clinical: HBIG is a sterile solution of immunoglobulin (10-18% protein) containing a high titer of antibody to hepatitis B surface antigen. It is most commonly used as prophylaxis therapy for infants born to hepatitis B surface antigen positive mothers. Its use in a breastfeeding mother would not harm a breastfeeding infant.

HEPATITIS B INFECTION;   *Hepatitis B Infection*

Uses: Hepatitis B exposure

AAP: Not reviewed

T½= ; **RID=** ; **Oral =** ; **MW=**

Clinical: Hepatitis B virus (HBV) causes a wide spectrum of infections, ranging from a mild asymptomatic form to a fulminant fatal hepatitis. Infants of mothers who are HBV positive (HBsAg) should be given Hepatitis immune globulin (HBIG) (preferably within 1 hour of birth) and a Hepatitis B vaccination AT BIRTH, which is believed to effectively reduce the risk of post-natal transmission, particularly via breastmilk.

HEPATITIS B VACCINE;   *Heptavax-B, Energix-B, Recombivax HB*   **L2**

Uses: Hepatitis B vaccination   **C**

AAP: Not reviewed

T½= ; **RID=** ; **Oral =** ; **MW=**

Clinical: Hepatitis B vaccine is an inactivated non-infectious hepatitis B surface antigen vaccine. It can be used in pediatric patients at birth. No data are available on its use in breastfeeding mothers, but it is unlikely to produce untoward effects on a breastfeeding infant. In infants born of HB surface antigen positive mothers, the American Academy of Pediatrics recommends hepatitis B vaccine (along with HBIG) should be administered to the infant within 1-12 hours of birth (0.5 mL IM) and again at 1 and 6 months. If so administered, breastfeeding poses no additional risk for acquisition of HBV by the infant.

HEPATITIS C INFECTION;   *Hepatitis C Infection, HCV*   **L2**

Uses: Hepatitis exposure

AAP: Not reviewed

T½= ; **RID=** ; **Oral =** ; **MW=**

Clinical: A number of studies have yet to document horizontal transmission of HCV to infant from their mothers breastmilk. Available data seem to suggest an elevated risk of vertical transmission to the infant occurs in HIV infected women and women with elevated titers of HCV RNA. The AAP recommends that HCV-infected women should be counseled that transmission of HCV by breastfeeding is theoretically possible but has not yet been documented. The Center for Disease Control (CDC) does not consider chronic hepatitis C infection in the mother as a contraindication to breastfeeding. All of the data thus far, clearly suggests that the horizontal transmission of HCV to a breastfeeding infant via breastmilk is remote and as yet unreported. However, it still may be prudent for mothers who are seropositive for HCV to abstain from breastfeeding if their nipples are cracked and bleeding.

HERBAL TEAS; *Herbal Teas*

Uses: Herbal teas, tablets, powders, antioxidants

AAP: Not reviewed

T½= ;   RID= ;   Oral = ;   MW=

Clinical: Herbal teas should be used with great caution, if at all. A number of reports in the literature indicate potential toxicity in pregnant women from some herbal teas which contain pyrrolizidine alkaloids (PA). Such alkaloids have been associated with feticide, birth defects and liver toxicity. Other hepatotoxic remedies include gerrymander, comfrey, mistletoe and skullcap, margosa oil, mate tea, Gordolobo yerba tea, and pennyroyal (squawmint) oil. A recent report of seven poisonings with anticholinergic symptoms following ingestion of "Paraguay Tea" was published and was an apparent adulteration. A recent report on Blue Cohosh suggests it is cardiotoxic when used late in pregnancy (see blue cohosh). Because exact ingredients are seldom listed on many teas, this author strongly suggests that lactating mothers limit exposure to these substances as much as possible. Never consume herbal remedies of unknown composition. Remember, breastfeeding infants are much more susceptible to such toxicants than are adults.

HEROIN; *Heroin*   L5

Uses: Narcotic analgesic   B

AAP: Drugs of abuse for which adverse effects have been reported

T½= 1.5-2 hours; **RID**= ; **Oral** = Poor; **MW**= 369

Clinical: Heroin is diacetyl-morphine (diamorphine), a prodrug that is rapidly converted to morphine. With oral use, rapid and complete first-pass metabolism occurs in the liver. Heavily dependent users should probably be advised against breastfeeding and their infants converted to formula. Heroin, as is morphine, is known to transfer into breastmilk. See morphine.

HERPES SIMPLEX INFECTIONS

Uses: Herpes simplex type I, II

AAP: Breastfeeding is acceptable if no lesions are on the breast or are adequately covered

T½= ; **RID**= ; **Oral** = ; **MW**=

Clinical: HSV-1 and HSV-2 have been isolated from human milk, even in the absence of vesicular lesions or drainage. Transmission after birth can occur and herpetic infections during the neonatal period are often severe and fatal. Exposure to the virus from skin lesions of caregivers, including lesions of the breast, have been described. Breastmilk does not appear to be a common mode of transmission although women with active lesions around the breast and nipple should refrain from breastfeeding until the lesions are adequately covered. Mothers with a lesion on one nipple, should breastfeed from the opposite side. A number of cases of herpes simplex transmission via breastmilk have been reported. Women with active lesions should be extremely meticulous in hand washing to prevent spread of the disease from other active lesions.

HEXACHLOROPHENE; *Septisol, Phisohex, Septi-Soft, pHisoHex, Sapoderm*   L4

Uses: Antiseptic scrub   C

AAP: Not reviewed

T½= ; **RID**= ; **Oral** = Complete; **MW**= 407

Clinical: Hexachlorophene is an antibacterial that is an effective inhibitor of gram positive organisms. It is generally used topically as a surgical scrub and sometimes vaginally in mothers. It has been implicated in causing brain lesions, blindness, and respiratory failure in both animals and humans. Although there are no studies reporting concentrations of this compound in breastmilk, it is probably transferred to some degree. Topical use in infants is absolutely discouraged due to the high absorption of hexachlorophene through an infant's skin and proven toxicity.

HIV INFECTION; *AIDS*	L5

Uses: Aids, HIV infections

AAP: Advise not to breastfeed

T½= ;   RID= ;   Oral = ;   MW=

Clinical: The AIDS (HIV) virus has been isolated from human milk. In addition, recent reports from throughout the world have documented the transmission of HIV through human milk. Women who develop a primary HIV infection while breastfeeding may shed especially high concentrations of HIV viruses and pose a high risk of transmission to their infants. Because the risk is now well documented, HIV infected mothers in the USA and others countries with safe alternative sources of feeding should be advised to not breastfeed their infants.

HUMAN IMMUNE GLOBULIN SUBCUTANEOUS; *Hizentra*	L2

Uses: Treatment of primary immunodeficiency | C

AAP: Not reviewed

T½= ;   RID= ;   Oral = ;   MW=

Clinical: Consists of human IgG. IgG transfer into human milk is negligible. No know risks to a breastfeeding infant.

HUMAN IMMUNE GLOBULIN; *Privigen*	L2

Uses: Treatment of primary immunodeficiency | C

AAP: Not reviewed

T½= ;   RID= ;   Oral = ;   MW=

Clinical: Consists of human IgG. IgG transfer into human milk is negligible. No know risks to a breastfeeding infant.

HYALURONIC ACID; *Synvisc, Euflexxa, Healon, Hyalgan, Hylaform, Juvederm, Orthovisc, Provisc, Restylane, Cystistat, Durolane, Eyestil, OrthoVisc, Suplasyn*	L3

Uses: Viscoelastic agent, antirheumatic, anti-wrinkle

AAP: Not reviewed

T½= ;   RID= ;   Oral = Nil;   MW= Large

Clinical: Large polymer of hyaluronic acid. Unlikely to enter milk. Unlikely to ever be orally bioavailable. Probably of no risk to a breastfed infant.

HYDRALAZINE; *Apresoline, Novo-Hylazin, Apo-Hydralazine*	L2
Uses: Antihypertensive	C
AAP: Maternal medication usually compatible with breastfeeding	
T½= 1.5-8 hours; **RID**= 1.2%; **Oral** = 30-50%; **MW**= 160	
Clinical: Hydralazine is a popular antihypertensive used for severe pre-eclampsia and gestational and postpartum hypertension. Levels in milk are far less than the pediatric clinical dose.	

HYDROCHLOROTHIAZIDE ; *HydroDIURIL, Esidrix, Oretic, Tekturna HCT, Apo-Hydro, Diuchlor H, Hydrodiuril, Novo-Hydrazide*	L2
Uses: Thiazide diuretic, antihypertensive	B
AAP: Maternal medication usually compatible with breastfeeding	
T½= 5.6-14.8 hours; **RID**= ; **Oral** = 72%; **MW**= 297	
Clinical: Hydrochlorothiazide (HCTZ) is a typical thiazide diuretic. The dose ingested (assuming milk intake of 600 mL) would be approximately 50 µg/day, a clinically insignificant amount. The concentration of HCTZ in the infant's serum was undetectable (<20 ng/mL). Most thiazide diuretics are considered compatible with breastfeeding if doses are kept low.	

HYDROCODONE; *Lortab, Vicodin, Maxidone, Norco, Hycodan, Robidone*	L3
Uses: Analgesic for pain	B
AAP: Not reviewed	
T½= 3.8 hours; **RID**= 3.1-3.7%; **Oral** = Complete; **MW**= 299	

Clinical: Hydrocodone is a narcotic analgesic and antitussive structurally related to codeine although somewhat more potent. It is commonly used in breastfeeding mothers throughout the USA. In a study of two breastfeeding women taking hydrocodone for various periods, patient one received a total of 63,525 μg (998.8 μg/kg) over 86.5 hours. Patient two, received 9075 μg (123.5 μg/kg) over 36 hours.

In patient one, the AUC of the drug concentration in milk was 4946.1 μg/L·hr and an average milk concentration of 57.2 μg/L. The authors estimate the relative infant dose at 3.1%. In patient two, the AUC of the drug concentration in milk was 735.6 μg/L·hr and an average milk concentration of 20.4 μg/L. The authors estimate the relative infant dose at 3.7%. This paper concluded that high doses of hydrocodone in mothers who are nursing newborn or premature infants can be concerning. Mothers should be advised to watch for sedation and appropriate weight gain in their infants.

HYDROCORTISONE ENEMA; *Colocort, Cortenema, Hycort Enema, Rectoid, Anucort, Proctosol*	L3
Uses: Corticosteroid	C
AAP: Not reviewed	

T½= 1-2 hours; **RID=** ; **Oral** = 96%; **MW=** 362

Clinical: Hydrocortisone administered rectally is probably okay if used short-term. Transfer into milk is probably low, although we have no data. No adverse effects have been reported in breastfed infants.

HYDROCORTISONE TOPICAL; *Westcort, Lipsovir, Cortate, Cortone, Emo-Cort, Aquacort*	L2
Uses: Corticosteroid	C
AAP: Not reviewed	

T½= 1-2 hours; **RID=** ; **Oral** = 96%; **MW=** 362

Clinical: Hydrocortisone administered topically is probably safe to use during breastfeeding. Transfer to milk is likely minimal. Topical application to the nipple is generally approved by most authorities if amounts applied and duration of use are minimized. Only small amounts should be applied and then only after feeding; larger quantities should be removed prior to breastfeeding.

HYDROMORPHONE; *Dilaudid, Exalgo, Hydromorph Contin*	L3
Uses: Opiate analgesic	C
AAP: Not reviewed	
T½= 11.1 hours; **RID=** 0.7%; **Oral** = 51%; **MW=** 285	

Clinical: Hydromorphone is a super potent morphine derivative. Reported milk levels following intranasal (2 mg) use are quite low averaging approximately 1 ug/mL over 24 hours. The relative infant dose is approximately 0.7. The clinical dose in milk is probably too low to affect an infant. However, high doses and prolonged usage could lead to sedation, just as with other opiates.

HYDROQUINONE; *Esoterica, Eldoquin, Melpaque, Melanex, Solaquin, Nuquin, Viquin*	L3
Uses: Depigmenting agent for topical applications	C
AAP: Not reviewed	
T½= ; **RID=** ; **Oral** = ; **MW=**	

Clinical: Well absorbed orally and through the skin. No data are available on its transfer into human milk. Although it is quite polar and water soluble, it also might be trapped in human milk. While it does not seem to be very toxic, its chronic use in breastfeeding mothers is probably not warranted for such benign syndromes that could wait until the mother has weaned.

HYDROXYCHLOROQUINE; *Plaquenil*	L2
Uses: Antimalarial, antirheumatic	C
AAP: Maternal medication usually compatible with breastfeeding	
T½= >40 days; **RID=** 2.9%; **Oral** = 74%; **MW=** 336	

Clinical: Milk levels are quite low. Huge volume of distribution which suggests milk levels are generally low.

HYDROXYUREA; *Hydrea*	L2
Uses: Antineoplastic agent	D
AAP: Not reviewed	
T½= 3-4 hours; **RID=** 4.3%; **Oral** = Complete; **MW=** 76	

Clinical: Well absorbed orally and rapidly metabolized to urea by the liver. Due to rapid metabolism, levels in milk are low.

HYDROXYZINE; *Atarax, Vistaril, Apo-Hydroxyzine, Novo-Hydroxyzin*	**L1**
Uses: Antihistamine, antiemetic	**C**

AAP: Not reviewed

T½= 3-7 hours; **RID=** ; **Oral** = Complete; **MW=** 375

Clinical: Hydroxyzine is an antihistamine structurally similar to cyclizine and meclizine. It produces significant CNS depression, anticholinergic side effects (drying), and antiemetic side effects. Hydroxyzine is largely metabolized to cetirizine (Zyrtec). No data are available on secretion into breastmilk.

HYLAN G-F 20; *Synvisc*	**L2**
Uses: Joint lubricant for arthritic pain	

AAP: Not reviewed

T½= ; **RID=** ; **Oral** = None; **MW=** 6 mil

Clinical: Hylan G-F 20 (Synvisc) is an elastoviscous fluid containing hylan polymers produced from chicken combs. Hylans are a natural complex sugar of the glycosaminoglycan family. Hylans are large molecular weight polymers and would not be expected to enter milk. Average molecular weight is 6 million daltons. This product would not pose a problem for a breastfeeding mother or infant.

HYOSCYAMINE; *Anaspaz, Levsin, NuLev*	**L3**
Uses: Anticholinergic, antisecretory agent	**C**

AAP: Not reviewed

T½= 3.5 hours; **RID=** ; **Oral** = 81%; **MW=** 289

Clinical: Hyoscyamine is an anticholinergic. Its typical effects are to dry secretions, produce constipation, dilate pupils, blur vision, and may produce urinary retention. Although no exact amounts are published, hyoscyamine is known to be secreted into breastmilk in trace amounts. Thus far, no untoward effects from breastfeeding while using hyoscyamine have been found. Caution.

I-125 I-131 I-123; *Radioactive Iodine, Iodine-125, Iodine-131, Iodine-123, Iodotope, I-125, I-131, I-123*	**L4**
Uses: Radioactive iodine	

AAP: Radioactive compound that requires temporary cessation of breastfeeding

T½= ;   **RID=** ;   **Oral** = Complete;   **MW=**

Clinical: The return to breastfeeding depends on the dose and the isotope used. It is most important with I-[131]. Radioiodine concentrates in milk where at least 26-45% of the dose ends up in the breast. Radiographs show major concentration in breastmilk. In scanning procedures where only a few microcuries are used (< 14 uCi), the mother may be able to return to breastfeeding within 20 days or perhaps less depending on the dose (see reference 5). In cases where ablation doses are used (300-700 mCi), the risk to the breastfeeding mother (breast cancer) is significant, and the risk to the infant is major (future thyroid cancer). We do not have data on how long the interruption should be following ablative doses, but it could be long (>>20 days). In all instances, simply counting the milk could provide the answer. However with ablative doses, it is probably advisable to discontinue breastfeeding, dry up, and then initiate treatment to try and avoid high exposure of breast tissue.

IBUPROFEN; *Advil, Nuprin, Motrin, Pediaprofen, Actiprofen, Amersol*	**L1**
Uses: Analgesic, antipyretic	**B**

AAP: Maternal medication usually compatible with breastfeeding

T½= 1.8-2.5 hours;   **RID=** 0.7%;   **Oral** = 80%;   **MW=** 206

Clinical: Ibuprofen is the ideal analgesic in breastfeeding mothers. It is secreted minimally into breast milk, almost undetectable. Commonly given to infants to alleviate fevers. No adverse effects are expected.

IFOSFAMIDE; *Holoxan, Ifex, Ifolem*	**L4**
Uses: Anti cancer agent	**D**

AAP: Not reviewed

T½= 7 to 15 hours;   **RID=** ;   **Oral** = 92% to 100%;   **MW=** 261

Clinical: Ifosfamide (IF) is structurally similar to Cyclophosphamide and is used in breast cancer. This family require activation(metabolism) by the liver to produce the active cytotoxic agents. The oral bioavailability of IF is near 100% and reaches a peak at 1-2 hours. IF is eliminated with a mono exponential curve. The elimination half-life (T½ beta) ranges from 3.8 to 8.6 hours. Active metabolites stay in the plasma compartment with brief half-lives of 4-6 hours or less. Transport of IF and its metabolites into the CNS is exceedingly low (approximately 1/6th of the plasma compartment). This would suggest milk levels will probably be low when they are ultimately determined. The kinetics of this agent are highly variable depending on the renal function, creatinine clearance, liver function, etc. Waiting periods before returning to breastfeeding should be adjusted for this factor. Withhold breastfeeding for at least 72 hours.

IMATINIB MESYLATE; *Gleevec*	L5
Uses: Antineoplastic agent, tyrosine kinase inhibitor	D
AAP: Not reviewed	
T½= 18 hours; **RID=** ; **Oral** = 98%; **MW**= 590	

Clinical: Imatinib is an anti-neoplastic agent used against gastrointestinal stromal tumors and various types of leukemia. Imatinib and its active metabolite are excreted into human milk. Based on data from three breastfeeding women taking Gleevec, the milk:plasma ratio is about 0.5 for imatinib and about 0.9 for the active metabolite. Considering the combined concentration of imatinib and active metabolite, a breastfed infant could receive up to 10 % of the maternal therapeutic dose based on body weight. Because of the potential for serious adverse reactions in nursing infants from Gleevec, a decision should be made whether to discontinue nursing or to discontinue the drug, taking into account the importance of the drug to the mother.

IMIPENEM-CILASTATIN; *Primaxin*	L2
Uses: Antibiotic	C
AAP: Not reviewed	
T½= 0.85-1.3 hours; **RID=** ; **Oral** = Poor; **MW**= 317	

Clinical: Imipenem is structurally similar to penicillins and acts similarly. Cilastatin is added to extend the half-life of imipenem. Both imipenem and cilastatin are poorly absorbed orally and must be administered IM or IV.[1,2] Imipenem is destroyed by gastric acidity. Transfer into breastmilk is probably minimal but no data are available. Changes in GI flora could occur but is probably remote.

IMIPRAMINE; *Tofranil, Janimine, Apo-Imipramine, Impril, Novo-Pramine*	L2
Uses: Tricyclic antidepressant	D

AAP: Drugs whose effect on nursing infants is unknown but may be of concern

T½= 8-16 hours; **RID=** 0.1% - 4.4%; **Oral =** 90%; **MW=** 280

Clinical: Imipramine is a classic tricyclic antidepressant. Imipramine is metabolized to desipramine, the active metabolite. Milk levels approximate those of maternal serum. Levels in milk are low. Probably compatible with breastfeeding.

INDAPAMIDE; *Lozol, Lozide, Gen-Indapamide, Apo-Indapamide*	L3
Uses: Antihypertensive diuretic	B

AAP: Not reviewed

T½= 14 hours; **RID=** ; **Oral =** Complete; **MW=** 366

Clinical: Indapamide is the first of a new class of indoline diuretics used to treat hypertension. No data exists on transfer into human milk. Some diuretics may reduce the production of breastmilk. See hydrochlorothiazide as alternative.

[111M] INDIUM; *[111]-Indium*	L4
Uses: Radioactive diagnostic agent	

AAP: Radioactive compound that requires temporary cessation of breastfeeding

T½= 2.8 days; **RID=** ; **Oral =** ; **MW=** 358

Clinical: [111]Indium is a radioactive material used for imaging neuroendocrine tumors. While the plasma half-life is extremely short (<10 minutes), with the majority of this product leaving the plasma compartment and distributing to tissue sites, the radioactive half-life is 2.8 days. In one patient receiving 12 MBq (0.32 mCi), the concentration in milk at 6 and 20 hours was 0.09 Bq/mL and 0.20 Bq/mL per MBq injected. These data indicate that breastfeeding may be safe if this radiopharmaceutical is used. Assuming an ingestion of 500 cc daily, the infant would receive approximately 100 Bq per MBq given to the mother (approximately 0.1 µCi). The NRC recommends a waiting period of 1 week with doses of 20 MBq (0.5 mCi), however see appendix B for current recommendations.

INDOMETHACIN; *Indocin, Apo-Indomethacin, Indocid, Novo-Methacin*	**L3**
Uses: Non-steroidal antiinflammatory	**B**

AAP: Maternal medication usually compatible with breastfeeding

T½= 4.5 hours; **RID=** 1.2%; **Oral =** 90%; **MW=** 357

Clinical: Indomethacin is a potent, nonsteroidal antiinflammatory agent frequently used in arthritis. It is also used in newborns in neonatal units to close a patent ductus arteriosus. There is one reported case of convulsions in an infant of a breastfeeding mother early postpartum (day 7). Infant dose is probably quite low.

INFLIXIMAB; *Remicade*	**L2**
Uses: Treatment of Crohn's, rheumatoid arthritis	**B**

AAP: Not reviewed

T½= 8-9.5 days; **RID=** ; **Oral =** Nil; **MW=** 149,100

Clinical: Large peptide and is probably unable to enter milk compartment. Would not be orally bioavailable. In a study of one breastfeeding patient who received 5 mg/kg IV, infliximab levels were determined in milk. None was detected in milk at any time (detection limit <0.1 µg/mL).

INFLUENZA VIRUS VACCINES; *Vaccine- Influenza, Flu-Imune, Fluogen, Fluzone, FluMist, Flu Vaccine, Agriflu, Fluarix, Fluviral*	**L1**
Uses: Vaccine	**C**

AAP: Not reviewed

T½= ; RID= ; Oral = ; MW=

Clinical: Inactivated intramuscular vaccines are approved for use in breastfeeding mothers by the CDC and the Academy of Pediatrics. FluMist (live attenuated virus) has not yet been studied or cleared for use in younger infants, although a number of studies suggest it is safe. At this time, the injectable form of influenza vaccine is preferred for breastfeeding mothers. The use of FluMist in breastfeeding mothers is yet to be studied. Due to its heat lability, the FluMist virus is unlikely to ever survive the plasma compartment nor the milk compartment, but this has yet to be studied.

INFLUENZA

Uses: Viral infection

AAP: Not reviewed

T½= ; RID= ; Oral = ; MW=

Clinical: Influenza is not a contraindication to breastfeeding. Breastfeeding has also been found to be beneficial in limiting the severity of respiratory infections in infants. Also, because the virus can be spread 24 to 48 hours prior to the onset of symptoms, the infant has been exposed to the virus prior to the mother knowing she has an infection.

INSECT STINGS;   *Insect Stings, Spider Stings, Bee Stings*

Uses: Insect stings, envenomations

AAP: Not reviewed

T½= ; RID= ; Oral = ; MW=

Clinical: Insect stings are primarily composed of small peptides, enzymes such as hyaluronidase, and other factors such as histamine. Because the total injectant is so small, most reactions are local. In cases of systemic reactions, the secondary release of maternal reactants produces the allergic response in the injected individual. Nevertheless, the amount of injection is exceedingly small. In the case of black widow spiders, the venom is so large in molecular weight (130 kDal for alpha-toxin), it would not likely penetrate milk. In addition, most of the venoms and allergens would be destroyed in the acidic milieu of the infant's stomach. The sting of the Loxosceles spider (brown recluse, fiddleback) is primarily a local necrosis without systemic effects. No report of toxicity to nursing infants has been reported from insect stings.

INSULIN GLARGINE; *Lantus*	L1
Uses: Long-acting recombinant insulin	C

AAP: Not reviewed

T½= 5-15 minutes; **RID=** ; **Oral** = None; **MW=** 6063

Clinical: Insulin glargine is insulin with slight changes in 3 amino acids. When injected subcutaneously, it precipitates into crystals that slows its absorption, thus this product works for about 24 hours. It would be largely destroyed in the GI tract of the infant and would produce virtually no oral absorption.

INSULIN; *Humulin, Novolin, Humalog, Iletin*	L1
Uses: Human insulin	B

AAP: Not reviewed

T½= ; **RID=** ; **Oral** = 0%; **MW=** >6000

Clinical: Insulin is a large peptide that is not secreted into milk. Even if secreted, it would be destroyed in the infant's GI tract leading to minimal or no absorption.

INTERFERON ALFA-2B; *PegIntron, Intron A*	L3
Uses: Anti viral	C

AAP: Not reviewed

T½= 2 to 3 hours ; **RID=** ; **Oral** = 80-90%; **MW=**

Clinical: Peginterferon alfa-2b is a pegylated form of the antiviral drug interferon alfa-2b. Pegylation confers protection against enzymatic degradation systemically. It is indicated for the treatment of hepatitis C. While we have no data on its use in breastfeeding mothers, other data on interferon's (alfa and beta) suggest they do not readily enter the milk, and milk levels will be exceeding low. When combined with ribavirin, breastfeeding is not recommended. Ribavirin is extremely teratogentic, do not use in pregnancy.

INTERFERON ALPHA-N3; *Alferon N, Interferon Alpha, PEG-Intron*	L2
Uses: Immune modulator, antiviral	C

AAP: Maternal medication usually compatible with breastfeeding

T½= 5-7 hours; **RID=** ; **Oral** = Low; **MW=** 28,000

Clinical: Very little is known about the secretion of interferons in human milk although some interferons are known to be secreted normally and may contribute to the antiviral properties of human milk. However, interferons are large in molecular weight (16-28,000 daltons), which would limit their transfer into human milk. In one study by the author virtually no interferon was transferred into human milk.

INTERFERON BETA-1A; *Avonex, Rebif*	L2
Uses: Immune modulator	C
AAP: Not reviewed	
T½= 10 Hours; RID= ; Oral = Minimal; MW= 22,500	

Clinical: Interferon beta-1a is probably safe to use during breastfeeding, and may be the preferred choice in patients with multiple sclerosis. Due to its exceedingly large molecular weight, transfer into milk is minimal. Interferons are generally nontoxic and used in large doses in infants clinically. In a study by the author, virtually none was transferred into human milk.

INTERFERON BETA-1B; *Betaseron, Extavia*	L2
Uses: Antiviral, immunomodulator	C
AAP: Not reviewed	
T½= 4.3 hours; RID= ; Oral = Poor; MW= 22,500	

Clinical: The transfer of interferon Beta-1a (Avonex, Rebif) is essentially nil and it is likely the same for this product, interferon Beta-1b. In a study by the author, virtually none was transferred into human milk.

IODINATED GLYCEROL; *Organidin, Iophen, R-GEN*	L4
Uses: Expectorant	X
AAP: Not reviewed	
T½= ; RID= ; Oral = Complete; MW= 258	

Clinical: This product contains 50% organically bound iodine. High levels of iodine are known to be secreted in milk. Milk/plasma ratios as high as 26 have been reported. Following absorption by the infant, high levels of iodine could lead to severe thyroid depression in infants. Normal iodine levels in breastmilk are already four times higher that RDA for infant. Expectorants, including iodine, work very poorly. Recently, many iodine containing products have been replaced with guaifenesin, which is considered safer. High levels of iodine-containing drugs should not be used in lactating mothers.

IPRATROPIUM BROMIDE; *Atrovent, Apo-Ipravent*	L2
Uses: Bronchodilator in asthmatics	B
AAP: Not reviewed	
T½= 2 hours; **RID=** ; **Oral =** 0-2%; **MW=** 412	

Clinical: Ipratropium is an anticholinergic drug that is used via inhalation for dilating the bronchi of asthmatics. Ipratropium is a quaternary ammonium compound, and although no data exists, it probably penetrates into breastmilk in exceedingly small levels due to its structure. It is unlikely that the infant would absorb any, due to the poor tissue distribution and oral absorption of this family of drugs.

IRBESARTAN; *Avapro, Avalide*	L3
Uses: Antihypertensive	C
AAP: Not reviewed	
T½= 11-15 hours; **RID=** ; **Oral =** 60-80%; **MW=** 428	

Clinical: Irbesartan is an angiotensin-II receptor antagonist used as an antihypertensive. Low concentrations are known to be secreted into rodent milk, but human studies are lacking. Both the ACE inhibitor family and the specific AT1 inhibitors such as irbesartan are contraindicated in the 2nd and 3rd trimesters of pregnancy due to severe hypotension, neonatal skull hypoplasia, irreversible renal failure, and death in the newborn infant. However, some of ACE inhibitors can be used in breastfeeding mothers postpartum. Some caution is recommended particularly with in mothers with premature infants.

IRON DEXTRAN; *INFeD*	L2
Uses: Iron supplement	C
AAP: Not reviewed	

T½= ; **RID**= ; **Oral** = ; **MW**=

Clinical: While there are no data available on the transfer of iron dextran into human milk, it is extremely unlikely due to its massive molecular weight. Further, iron is transferred into human milk by a tightly controlled pumping system that first chelates the iron to a high molecular weight protein and then transfers it into the milk compartment. It is generally well known that dietary supplements of iron do not change milk levels of iron significantly.

IRON SUCROSE; *Venofer*	L3
Uses: Iron supplement	B
AAP: Not reviewed	

T½= 6 hours; **RID**= ; **Oral** = Poor; **MW**= 34,000-60,000

Clinical: Iron sucrose is used in the treatment of iron-deficiency anemia in chronic renal failure. Once dissociated, the iron is incorporated into hemoglobin. There have been no studies of the secretion of iron sucrose in human milk. This product is a polymerized form of polynuclear iron (III)-hydroxide in sucrose. Used intravenously, it is sequestered in the liver where it is metabolized and free iron is released into the circulation. Due to its size, it is unlikely to enter mature milk.

IRON; *Fer-In-Sol, Infufer, Jectofer, Slow-Fe*	L1
Uses: Metal supplement	
AAP: Not reviewed	

T½= ; **RID**= ; **Oral** = <30%; **MW**= 56

Clinical: The secretion of iron salts into breastmilk appears to be very low although the bioavailability of that present in milk is high. One recent study suggests that supplementation is not generally required until the 4th month postpartum when some breastfed infants may become iron deficient although these assumptions are controversial. Premature infants are more susceptible to iron deficiencies because they do not have the same hepatic stores available as full term infants. These authors recommend iron supplementation, particularly in exclusively breastfed infants, beginning at 4th month. Supplementation in pre-term infants should probably be initiated earlier. However, oral supplemental iron may block some of the antibacterial properties of human milk. The use of relatively high doses in breastfeeding mothers is probably not contraindicated, due to the fact that iron transports very poorly to the milk compartment.

ISOETHARINE; *Bronkosol, Bronkometer*	L2

Uses: Bronchodilator	C

AAP: Not reviewed

T½= 1-3 hours; **RID=** ; **Oral =** ; **MW=** 239

Clinical: Isoetharine is a selective beta-2 adrenergic bronchodilator for asthmatics. There are no reports on its secretion into human milk.   However, plasma levels following inhalation are exceedingly low, and breastmilk levels would similarly be low. Isoetharine is rapidly metabolized in the GI tract, so oral absorption by the infant would likely be minimal.

ISOMETHEPTENE MUCATE; *Midrin*	L3

Uses: For tension and migraine headache	

AAP: Not reviewed

T½= ; **RID=** ; **Oral =** ; **MW=** 493

Clinical: Isometheptene is a mild stimulate (sympathomimetic) that apparently acts by constricting dilated cranial and cerebral arterioles, thus reducing vascular headaches. It is listed as possibly effective by the FDA and is probably only marginally effective.   Midrin also contains acetaminophen and a mild sedative dichloralphenazone, of which little is known. No data are available on transfer into human milk. Due to its size and molecular composition, it is likely to attain low to moderate levels in breastmilk. Because better drugs exist for migraine therapy, this product is probably not a good choice for breastfeeding mothers. See sumatriptan, amitriptyline, or propranolol as alternatives.

ISONIAZID; *INH, Laniazid, Isotamine, PMS Isoniazid*	L3

Uses: Antituberculosis agent	C

AAP: Maternal medication usually compatible with breastfeeding

T½= 1.1 - 3.1 hours; **RID=** 1.2% - 18%; **Oral =** Complete; **MW=** 137

Clinical: Transfer of isoniazid into human milk is highly variable, close monitoring for liver toxicity and neuritis is advised. Breastfeeding immediately before taking isoniazid will allow infants to avoid peak concentrations at 1-2 hours after administration. Observe for fatigue, weakness, anorexia, nausea, and vomiting in the breastfed infant. AAP rates isoniazid as a medication usually compatible with breastfeeding. Suggest the mom breastfeed and then take isoniazid in an attempt to avoid the Cmax (peak) at 1-2 hours.

ISOPROTERENOL; *Medihaler-Iso, Isuprel, Medihaler-Iso*	L2
Uses: Bronchodilator	C
AAP: Not reviewed	

T½= 1-2 hours; **RID**= ; **Oral** = Poor; **MW**= 211

Clinical: Isoproterenol is an old adrenergic bronchodilator. Currently it is seldom used for this purpose. There are no data available on breastmilk levels. It is probably secreted into milk in extremely small levels. Isoproterenol is rapidly metabolized in the gut, and it is unlikely a breastfeeding infant would absorb clinically significant levels.

ISOSORBIDE DINITRATE; *Angidil, Angipec, Dilatate, Isordil, Apo-ISDN, Coronex, Coradur, Apo-ISDN*	L3
Uses: Vasodilating agents	C
AAP: Not reviewed	

T½= 5 hours (metabolite); **RID**= ; **Oral** = 10-90%; **MW**=

Clinical: The use of organic nitrates such as isosorbide dinitrate in breastfeeding mothers is potentially risky. We have no data on its transfer into human milk at all. It is rather small in molecular weight and could potentially end up in milk to some degree. I think it is unlikely the amount in milk would seriously impact a breastfeeding infant but this is only supposition.

ISOSORBIDE MONONITRATE; *Imdur, Coronex*	L3
Uses: Vasodilating agent	C
AAP: Not reviewed	

T½= 6.2 hours; **RID**= ; **Oral** = 93%; **MW**=

Clinical: The use of organic nitrates such as isosorbide mononitrate in breastfeeding mothers is potentially risky. We have no data on its transfer into human milk at all. It is rather small in molecular weight and could potentially end up in milk to some degree. I thinik it is unlikely the amount in milk would seriously impact a breastfeeding infant but this is only supposition.

ISOSULFAN BLUE; *Lymphazurin*	L4
Uses: Contrast agent	C

AAP: Not reviewed

T½= ; **RID=** ; **Oral** = ; **MW=** 566.7

Clinical: Isosulfan blue is a contrast agent used for visualization of the lymphatic system draining. No data has been reported on the transfer of isosulfan blue into breast milk, and therefore caution should be used in breastfeeding mothers.

ISOTRETINOIN; *Accutane, Isotrex*	L5
Uses: Vitamin A derivative used for acne	X

AAP: Not reviewed

T½= >20 hours; **RID=** ; **Oral** = 25%; **MW=** 300

Clinical: Isotretinoin is contraindicated for use in breastfeeding. It is highly lipophilic and concentrates in the milk. Use of isotretinoin during breastfeeding poses significant risk.

ISRADIPINE; *DynaCirc*	L3
Uses: Calcium channel blocker, antihypertensive	C

AAP: Not reviewed

T½= 8 hours; **RID=** ; **Oral** = 17%; **MW=** 371

Clinical: It is not known if isradipine is secreted into milk. However, other calcium channel blockers are transferred only minimally (see verapamil, nifedipine). Observe for lethargy, low blood pressure, and headache. See verapamil or nifedipine as alternatives.

ITRACONAZOLE; *Sporanox*	L2
Uses: Antifungal	C

AAP: Not reviewed

T½= 64 hours; **RID**= 0.2%; **Oral** = 55%; **MW**= 706

Clinical: Transfer of itraconazole into milk is minimal, and it is probably safe to use during pregnancy. Do not use with terfenadine and astemizole. The preferred antifungal in breastfeeding is fluconazole. No adverse effects have been reported in breastfed infants.

IVERMECTIN; *Mectizan*	L3
Uses: Antiparasitic	C

AAP: Maternal medication usually compatible with breastfeeding

T½= 28 hours; **RID**= 1.3%; **Oral** = Variable; **MW**=

Clinical: Ivermectin is now widely used to treat human worm infections. In one study, the average daily ingestion of ivermectin was calculated at 2.1 µg/kg which is 10 fold less than the adult dose. No adverse effects were reported.

KANAMYCIN; *Kantrex*	L2
Uses: Antibiotic	D

AAP: Maternal medication usually compatible with breastfeeding

T½= 2.4 hours; **RID**= 0.3%; **Oral** = 1%; **MW**=

Clinical: Kanamycin is an aminoglycoside antibiotic primarily used for gram negative infections. Levels in milk are low and the poor oral absorption (only 1%) in the infant would limit amount absorbed. Changes in GI flora are possible.

KAOLIN - PECTIN; *Kaolin, Kaopectate, Donnagel-MB, Kao-Con*	L1
Uses: Antidiarrhea	C

AAP: Not reviewed

T½= ; **RID**= ; **Oral** = 0%; **MW**=

Clinical: Kaolin-pectin is safe to use during breastfeeding, oral absorption is minimal. Some formulations may contain opiates, be advised. Observe for constipation.

KAVA-KAVA; *Awa, Kew, Tonga*	L5
Uses: Sedative and sleep enhancement	

AAP: Not reviewed

T½= ; RID= ; Oral = ; MW=

Clinical: Kava-Kava is contraindicated in breastfeeding. There are many harmful adverse effects associated with usage, mainly to the mother. The German Commission E monographs state that it is contraindicated in pregnant and lactating women.

KETAMINE; *Ketanest, Ketaset, Ketalar, Ketanest S, Ketamax, Calypsol, Brevinaze, Anesject*	**L3**
Uses: Anesthetic agent	**B**

AAP: Not reviewed

T½= 2.5-3 hours; **RID**= ; **Oral** = 16%; **MW**= 237

Clinical: Ketamine is a strong anesthetic agent that is used intranasally, intravenously, intramuscularly, and orally. Although we do not have levels in human milk, due to the rapid redistribution phase (4.68 minutes), milk levels will likely be small to nil after a few hours. Ketamine has a shorter half-life in children than in adults. Milk levels are likely to be low.

KETOCONAZOLE; *Nizoral Shampoo, Nizoral*	**L2**
Uses: Antifungal, anti-dandruff	**C**

AAP: Maternal medication usually compatible with breastfeeding

T½= 2-8 hours; **RID**= 0.3%; **Oral** = Variable (75%); **MW**= 531

Clinical: Ketoconazole is an antifungal similar in structure to miconazole and clotrimazole. It is used orally, topically, and via shampoo. Ketoconazole is not detected in plasma after chronic shampooing. Ketoconazole is probably safe in breastfeeding infants.

KETOPROFEN; *Orudis, Oruvail, Actron, Apo-Keto, Rhodis, Rhovail*	**L2**
Uses: NSAID analgesic	**B**

AAP: Not reviewed

T½= 2-4 hours; **RID**= 0.3%; **Oral** = 90%; **MW**= 254

Clinical: Ketoprofen is a typical nonsteroidal analgesic. It is structurally similar to ibuprofen. In one study, the mean and maximum doses that a breastfed newborn would ingest during one day is 7.0 and 9.0 µg/kg/day or about 0.3% of the weight-adjusted maternal dose. The authors suggest that breastfeeding is permissible when ketoprofen is administered to the mother to treat postpartum pain.

KETOROLAC TROMETHAMINE; *Sprix, Acuvail*	L3
Uses: Intranasal analgesic for acute moderate to severe pain	C/D
AAP: Not reviewed	
T½= ; **RID=** ; **Oral =** ; **MW=**	
Clinical: Ketorolac orally has been studied and levels in milk are low. This NSAID is probably safe for breastfeeding mothers and breastfeeding infants.	

KETOROLAC; *Toradol, Acular*	L2
Uses: Non-steroidal antiinflammatory, analgesic	C
AAP: Maternal medication usually compatible with breastfeeding	
T½= 2.4-8.6 hours; **RID=** 0.2%; **Oral =** >81%; **MW=** 255	
Clinical: Ketorolac is a popular, nonsteroidal analgesic. Although previously used in labor and delivery, its use has subsequently been contraindicated because it is believed to adversely effect fetal circulation and inhibit uterine contractions, thus increasing the risk of hemorrhage. However, levels in milk are incredibly low and it is probably safe to use in breastfeeding mothers.	

KOMBUCHA TEA	L5
Uses: Herbal tea	
AAP: Not reviewed	
T½= ; **RID=** ; **Oral =** ; **MW=**	
Clinical: Kombucha tea is a popular health beverage made by incubating the Kombucha mushroom in sweet black tea. During 1995, several reported cases of toxicity and one fatality were reported to the CDC. Based on these reports, the Iowa Department of Health has recommended that persons refrain from drinking Kombucha tea until the role of the tea in these cases has been resolved.	

L-METHYLFOLATE; *Deplin, Metafolin*	L3
Uses: Active folic acid metabolite	
AAP: Not reviewed	
T½= ; **RID=** ; **Oral =** Complete; **MW=** 455	

Clinical: Use with caution in seizure patients, as levels of anticonvulsants may be reduced with this drug. However, this drug is unlikely to elevate milk folate levels. Several studies suggest that maternal supplementation with folic acid did not dramatically increase milk folate levels. This suggests that even following supplementation, milk levels would be unlikely to increase, unless the mother is deficient. Thus, this product is probably not hazardous to use in a breastfeeding mother.

LABETALOL; *Trandate, Normodyne*	L2

Uses: Antihypertensive, beta blocker	C

AAP: Maternal medication usually compatible with breastfeeding

T½= 6-8 hours; **RID=** 0.2% - 0.6%; **Oral =** 30-40%; **MW=** 328

Clinical: Labetalol is a selective beta blocker with moderate lipid solubility that is used as an antihypertensive and for treating angina. In one study levels in milk were extremely low, therefore, only small amounts are secreted into human milk.

LACOSAMIDE; *Vimpat*	L3

Uses: Anticonvulsant	C

AAP: Not reviewed

T½= 13 hours; **RID=** ; **Oral =** Complete; **MW=** 250

Clinical: Lacosamide is a new anticonvulsant used as adjunctive therapy in the treatment of partial-onset seizures in patients with epilepsy aged 17 years and older. It is a functionalized amino acid that has activity in the maximal electroshock seizure test. Due to its structure, levels in milk may be significant. No data are available on its transfer into human milk, but caution is recommended until we have more data.

LAMIVUDINE; *Epivir-HBV, 3TC, 3TC*	L2

Uses: Antiviral	C

AAP: Not reviewed

T½= 5-7 hours; **RID=** 4.3%; **Oral =** 82%; **MW=** 229

Clinical: Two studies now show that while the levels of lamivudine in milk are three times the maternal plasma levels, the serum levels in infants is far subclinical (10 fold). The concentration of lamivudine in milk is 1.8 mg/liter, thus an infant would only receive about 1 mg per day via milk. The standard antiretroviral dose in infants is 4 mg/kg/day, far more than is received via milk. This data suggests that the serum levels of lamivudine attained in the infant are probably too low to produce side effects in the infant, and certainly too low to treat HIV effectively.

LAMOTRIGINE; *Lamictal, Lamictal XR*	L3
Uses: Anticonvulsant	C

AAP: Drugs whose effect on nursing infants is unknown but may be of concern

T½= 29 hours; **RID=** 9.2% - 18.3%; **Oral** = 98%; **MW=** 256

Clinical: High relative infant dose and significantly high infant plasma levels (<=45% of maternal levels) suggests significant transfer to the infant. Infants should be closely monitored with occassional plasma levels. One case of severe apnea has been recently reported in a 16 day old breastfed infant. In this case, the mother was receiving 850 mg/day, had a plasma level of 14.93 µg/mL. The plasma level of the infant was 4.87 µg/mL. The use of lamotrigine in breastfeeding mothers produces significant plasma levels in some breastfed infants, although they are apparently not high enough to produce side effects in most cases. Exposure in utero is considerably higher, and levels will probably drop in newborn breastfed infants who are breastfed. Nevertheless, it is advisable to monitor the infant's plasma levels closely to insure safety.

LANSOPRAZOLE; *Prevacid, Prevpac, Prevacid NapraPak*	L3
Uses: Reduces stomach acid secretion	B

AAP: Not reviewed

T½= 1.5 hours; **RID=** ; **Oral** = 80% (Enteric only); **MW=** 369

Clinical: We have no data on the transfer of lansoprazole into human milk, but it is likely low. Other proton pump inhibitors like omeprazole are safe with minimal transfer to milk. Lansoprazole is probably safe. There should not be any severe adverse effects, possibly reduced stomach acidity in the infant.

LATANOPROST; *Xalatan*	L3
Uses: Prostaglandin for glaucoma	C

AAP: Not reviewed

T½= <30 minutes; **RID=** ; **Oral** = Nil; **MW=**

Clinical: Latanoprost is a prostaglandin F2-alpha analogue used for the treatment of ocular hypertension and glaucoma. One drop used daily is usually effective. No data are available on the transfer of this product into human milk, but it is unlikely. Prostaglandins are by nature, rapidly metabolized. Plasma levels are barely detectable and then only for 1 hour after use. Combined with the short half-life, minimal plasma levels, and poor oral bioavailability, untoward effects via milk are unlikely.

LEAD	L5
Uses: Environmental pollutant	

AAP: Not reviewed

T½= 20-30 years (bone); **RID=** ; **Oral** = 5-10%; **MW=** 207

Clinical: Lead is an environmental pollutant. It serves no useful purpose in the body and tends to accumulate in the body's bony structures based on their exposure. Due to the rapid development of the nervous system, children are particularly sensitive to elevated levels. Lead poisoning is known to significantly alter IQ and neuropsychologic development, particularly in infants. Therefore, infants receiving breastmilk from mothers with high lead levels should be closely monitored, and both mother and infant may require chelation and the infant transferred to formula. Depending on the choice of chelator, mothers undergoing chelation therapy to remove lead may mobilize significant quantities of lead and should not breastfeed during the treatment period unless the chelator is Succimer.

LEFLUNOMIDE; *Arava*	L4
Uses: Antimetabolite anti-inflammatory	X

AAP: Not reviewed

T½= >15-18 hours; **RID=** ; **Oral** = 80%; **MW=** 270

Clinical: Leflunomide is a new anti-inflammatory agent used for arthritis. It is an immunosuppressant that reduces pyrimidine synthesis. Leflunomide is metabolized to the active metabolite referred to as M1, which has a long half-life and slow elimination. This product is a potent immunosuppressant with a potential elevated risk of malignancy and teratogenicity in pregnant women. It is not known if it transfers into human milk, but use of this product while breastfeeding would be highly risky.

LEPIRUDIN; *Refludan*	L2
Uses: Thrombin inhibitor, anticoagulant	B
AAP: Not reviewed	

T½= 1.3 hours; **RID**= ; **Oral** = Nil; **MW**= 6979

Clinical: Large protein. Undetectable in one patient breastmilk sample following use. Unlikely it would be orally bioavailable.

LETROZOLE; *Femara*	L4
Uses: Aromatase inhibitor of estrogen synthesis	D
AAP: Not reviewed	

T½= 48 hours; **RID**= ; **Oral** = 90%; **MW**= 285

Clinical: Letrozole is an aromatase inhibitor of estrogen synthesis and is used to treat estrogen-receptor positive breast cancer and other syndromes. No data are available on its transfer to human milk but I would suspect the levels are low. However, it has a very long half-life which is concerning in a breastfed infant and could lead to higher plasma levels over time. Therefore, the transfer of small amounts of this agent to an infant could seriously impair bone growth or sexual development of an infant and for this reason it is probably somewhat hazardous to use in a breastfeeding mother.

LEUPROLIDE ACETATE; *Lupron, Viadur*	L5
Uses: Gonadotropin-Releasing hormone analog	X
AAP: Not reviewed	

T½= 3.6 hours; **RID**= ; **Oral** = None; **MW**= 1400

Clinical: It is not known whether leuprolide transfers into human milk, but due to its nonapeptide structure, it is not likely that its transfer would be extensive. In addition, animal studies have found that it has zero oral bioavailability; therefore, it is unlikely it would be orally bioavailable in the human infant if ingested via milk. Its effect on lactation is unknown, but it could suppress lactation particularly early postpartum. It is of no risk to the breastfed infant, only to milk production.

LEVALBUTEROL; *Xopenex*	**L2**
Uses: Bronchodilator	C

AAP: Not reviewed

T½= 3.3 hours; **RID**= ; **Oral** = 100%; **MW**= 275

Clinical: Levalbuterol is the active (R)-enantiomer of the drug substance racemic albuterol. It is a popular and new bronchodilator used in asthmatics. No data are available on breastmilk levels. After inhalation, plasma levels are incredibly low averaging 1.1 nanogram/mL. It is very unlikely that enough would enter milk to produce clinical effects in an infant. This product is commonly used in infancy for asthma and other bronchoconstrictive illnesses.

LEVETIRACETAM; *Keppra*	**L3**
Uses: Anticonvulsant	C

AAP: Not reviewed

T½= 6-8 hours; **RID**= 3.4% - 7.8%; **Oral** = 100%; **MW**= 170

Clinical: Levetiracetam is growing in popularity for the treatment of partial seizures, and has good absorption, distribution, and other pharmacokinetics. Maternal milk levels averaged 74 uM (12.6 mg/L). The relative infant dose reported was 5.5%. Most interesting was that the plasma levels in all the infants fell significantly following delivery, suggesting that far more is transferred in utero than via milk and that infants can clear it very quickly. No adverse effects were noted in any of the breastfeeding infants. The authors suggested that levetiracetam levels in breastfed infants are low.

LEVOBUNOLOL; *Bunolol, Betagan, Ophtho-Bunolol*	**L3**
Uses: Beta blocker for glaucoma	C

AAP: Not reviewed

T½= 6.1 hours; **RID**= ; **Oral** = Complete; **MW**= 291

Clinical: Levobunolol is a typical beta blocker used ophthalmically for treatment of glaucoma. Some absorption has been reported, with resultant bradycardia in patients. No data on transfer to human milk are available.

LEVOCABASTINE; *Livostin*	L2
Uses: Ophthalmic antihistamine for itching	C

AAP: Not reviewed

T½= 33-40 hours; **RID**= ; **Oral** = 100%; **MW**=

Clinical: Levocabastine is an antihistamine primarily used via nasal spray and eye drops. It is used for allergic rhinitis and ophthalmic allergies. After application to eye or nose, very low levels are attained in the systemic circulation (<1 ng/mL). In one nursing mother, it was calculated that the daily dose of levocabastine in the infant was about 0.5 µg, far too low to be clinically relevant.

LEVOCARNITINE; *Carnitor, Carnitor SF*	L3
Uses: Dietary Supplement	B

AAP: Not reviewed

T½= 17.4 hours; **RID**= ; **Oral** = 10-20%; **MW**= 161

Clinical: Levocarnitine is not overtly hazardous and is a normal biological factor required in humans. Levocarnitine supplements carnitine, a natural metabolic compound that facilitates the transfer of fatty acids into the mitochondria, thus ensuring energy production. A deficiency can be associated with excess acyl CoA esters and disruption of intermediary metabolism. Supplementation has not been studied in nursing mothers but it not likely hazardous.

LEVOCETIRIZINE; *Xyzal*	L3
Uses: Antihistamine	B

AAP: Not reviewed

T½= 8 hours ; **RID**= ; **Oral** = Complete; **MW**= 389

Clinical: Levocetirizine is a non-sedating antihistamine that is probably safe to use during breastfeeding. No data on the transfer into human milk are available at this time. Just as with cetirizine, it is probably compatible with breastfeeding.

LEVODOPA; *Dopar, Larodopa, Sinemet, Prolopa, Endo Levodopa/Carbidopa*	L4
Uses: Antiparkinsonian	C

AAP: Not reviewed

T½= 1-3 hours; **RID=** 1.7%; **Oral =** 41%-70%; **MW=** 197

Clinical: Observe for reduction of prolactin and milk synthesis. Milk levels appear too low to affect a breastfed infant. In one study dose to infant was small, only 23 ug/kg/d.No adverse reactions were noted in the breastfed infant, as the ingested amount was subtherapeutic.

Warning: Levodopa is known to suppress prolactin production in normal, and breastfeeding mothers. In one group of 6 postpartum women (2-4 days), levodopa suppressed basal serum prolactin levels by as much as 78%.

LEVOFLOXACIN; *Levaquin, Quixin*	L3
Uses: Fluoroquinolone antibiotic	C

AAP: Not reviewed

T½= 6-8 hours; **RID=** 10.5% - 17.2%; **Oral =** 99%; **MW=** 370

Clinical: Levofloxacin is a potent fluoroquinolone. This study was somewhat poorly done. While the peak levels were reported to be 8.2 ug/mL, the average milk level reported was 5 ug/mL. Using this data, the relative infant dose would range from 10.5% to 17%. However, the time-to-peak interval reported in this case was 5 hours, rather than 1-1.8 hours reported following both oral and IV doses in the prescribing information. Of the 10 reported levels in this study, only 1 was above 5 ug/mL. Thus the reported average level of 5 ug/mL is probably consistent with other data. This suggests a Milk/Plasma ratio of approximately 0.95 which is probably correct. Thus, levofloxacin concentrations in milk peak around 1-1.8 hours and at levels close to plasma levels. Observe the infant for changes in gut flora, candida overgrowth, or diarrhea.

LEVONORGESTREL (Plan B); *Plan B*	L2
Uses: Emergency contraceptive	X

AAP: Not reviewed

T½= 11-45; **RID=** ; **Oral =** Complete; **MW=** 312

Clinical: Levonorgestrel as a progestin is of limited risks to most breastfeeding mothers. This drug could potentially suppress milk production in some mothers. Nursing mothers who use relatively high doses of levonorgestrel are recommended to discontinue nursing for at least 8 hours post dose, and should resume feeding within 24 hours.

LEVONORGESTREL + ETHINYL ESTRADIOL; *Preven*	L3
Uses: Emergency contraceptive	X
AAP: Not reviewed	
T½= ; **RID=** ; **Oral =** ; **MW=**	

Clinical: Levonorgestrel and ethinyl estradiol (Preven) can be used as an emergency contraceptive. It is believed to act by preventing ovulation or fertilization by altering tubal transport of sperm and/or ova. It may as well partially inhibit implantation by altering the endometrium. For more details on each ingredient see their individual monographs. It should not be used in known or suspected pregnancy, in patients with pulmonary edema, ischemic heart disease, deep vein thrombosis, etc. The initial treatment of 2 tablets should be administered as soon as possible but within 72 hours of unprotected intercourse. This is followed by the second dose of 2 tablets 12 hours later. Because of its estrogen content, it may suppress milk production.

LEVONORGESTREL; *Norplant, Seasonale, Mirena IUD, Next Choice, Plan B One-Step*	L2
Uses: Implantable, oral, and intrauterine contraceptive	X
AAP: Maternal medication usually compatible with breastfeeding	
T½= 24 hours; **RID=** ; **Oral =** Complete; **MW=** 312	

Clinical: Levonorgestrel as a progestin is of limited risks to most breastfeeding mothers. However, when estrogens are added, the product becomes quite risky. Some mothers may report reduced milk production. No or little risk of sexual side effects in infants. As with any progestin or estrogen, observe for changes in milk productin.

LEVOTHYROXINE; *Synthroid, Levothroid, Unithroid, Eltroxin, Levoxyl, Thyroid, Levoxyl, Eltroxin*	L1
Uses: Thyroid supplements	A
AAP: Maternal medication usually compatible with breastfeeding	

T½= 6-7 days; **RID=** ; **Oral** = 50-80%; **MW=** 798

Clinical: Levothyroxine is also called T4. Most studies indicate that minimal levels of maternal thyroid are transferred into human milk, and further, that the amount secreted is extremely low and insufficient to protect a hypothyroid infant even while nursing. It is generally recognized that some thyroxine will transfer but the amount will be extremely low.

LIDOCAINE; *Xylocaine, Xylocard*	L2
Uses: Local anesthetic	B

AAP: Maternal medication usually compatible with breastfeeding

T½= 1.8 hours; **RID=** 0.5% - 3.1%; **Oral** = <35%; **MW=** 234

Clinical: There have been many studies done on the transfer of lidocaine into breast milk. All conclude that lidocaine transfer to milk is minimal and probably safe to use during breastfeeding. Dental procedure lidocaine usage is minimal and should pose no harm to the breastfed infant. Maternal plasma and milk levels do not seem to approach high concentrations and the oral bioavailability in the infant would be quite low (<35%).

LINCOMYCIN; *Lincocin*	L2
Uses: Antibiotic	C

AAP: Not reviewed

T½= 4.4-6.4 hours; **RID=** 0.7%; **Oral** = <30%; **MW=** 407

Clinical: Lincomycin is an effective antimicrobial used for gram positive and anaerobic infections. It is secreted into breastmilk in small but detectable levels. In a group of 9 mothers breastmilk concentrations ranged from 0.5 to 2.4 mg/L (mean= 1.28). Although effects on infant are unlikely, some modification of gut flora or diarrhea is possible.

LINDANE; *Kwell, G-well, Scabene, Hexit, Kwellada, PMS-Lindane*	L4
Uses: Pediculicide, scabicide	B

AAP: Not reviewed

T½= 18-21 hours; **RID=** ; **Oral** = ; **MW=** 290

Clinical: Lindane is an older pesticide also called gamma benzene hexachloride. It is primarily indicated for treatment of pediculus capitis (head lice) and less so for scabies (crab lice).   If used in children, lindane should not be left on the skin for more than 6 hours before being wash off as peak plasma levels occur in children at about 6 hours after application. Although there are reports of some resistance, head lice and scabies should generally be treated with permethrin products (NIX, Elimite), which are much safer in pediatric patients. See permethrin.

LINEZOLID; *Zyvox, Zyvoxam, Zyvoxid*	L3
Uses: Antibiotic	C

AAP: Not reviewed

T½= 5.2 hours; **RID=** ; **Oral** = 100%; **MW=** 337

Clinical: Linezolid is one of the newest antibiotics used to treat serious MRSA infections. At present we have no published levels in human milk, but levels will likely be low to negligible. Its use in children has expanded recently and clearance is actually higher in children than adults or infants. Side effects are minimal with this product. Recent studies have shown it quite safe for use in children and infants with minimal side effects, although it still does not have FDA clearance for children and infants. Use in breastfeeding mothers is unlikely to cause problems.

LIOTHYRONINE; *Cytomel*	L2
Uses: Thyroid supplement	A

AAP: Not reviewed

T½= 25 hours; **RID=** ; **Oral** = 95 %; **MW=** 651

Clinical: Liothyronine is also called T3. It is seldom used for thyroid replacement therapy due to its short half-life. It is generally recognized that only minimal levels of thyroid hormones are secreted in human milk although several studies have shown that hypothyroid conditions only became apparent when breastfeeding was discontinued. Although some studies indicate that breastfeeding may briefly protect hypothyroid infants, it is apparent that the levels of T4 and T3 are too low to provide long-term protection from hypothyroid disease. From severale studies, it is apparent that only exceedingly low levels of T3 are secreted into human milk and are insufficient to protect an infant from hypothyroidism.

LISINOPRIL; *Prinivil, Zestril, Apo-Lisinopril*	L3
Uses: Antihypertensive, ACE inhibitor	C

T½= 12 hours; **RID=** ; **Oral** = 29%; **MW=** 442

AAP: Not reviewed

Clinical: We have no data on lisinopril transfer into milk. Other ACE inhibitors such as enalapril are probably safe to use during breastfeeding and transfer is minimal. Monitor premature infants for renal toxicity. Otherwise, monitor for hypotension and weakness.

LITHIUM CARBONATE; *Lithobid, Eskalith, Carbolith, Duralith, Lithane*	L3
Uses: Antimanic drug in bipolar disorders	D

AAP: Drugs associated with significant side effects and should be given with caution

T½= 17-24 hours; **RID=** 12% - 30.1%; **Oral** = Complete; **MW=** 74

Clinical: Lithium readily transfers to the infant via milk. Infant plasma levels can be significant. If closely followed, most infants could continue to breastfeed, but close followup by attending physicians is mandatory. If the infant continues to breastfeed, it is strongly suggested that the infant be closely monitored for serum lithium levels, and BUN/Creatinine after 6 weeks or so. Levels drawn too early (7 days) may only reflect in utero exposure. A number of studies of lithium suggest that lithium administration is not an absolute contraindication to breastfeeding, if the physician monitors the infant closely for elevated plasma lithium. Current studies, as well as unpublished experience, suggest that the infant's plasma levels rise to about 30-40% of the maternal level, most often without untoward effects in the infant. Use with great caution and only with medical support.

LOMEFLOXACIN; *Maxaquin*	L3
Uses: Fluoroquinolone antibiotic	C

AAP: Not reviewed

T½= 8 hours; **RID=** ; **Oral** = 92%; **MW=** 351

Clinical: Lomefloxacin belongs the fluoroquinolone family of antimicrobials. At least one case of bloody colitis (pseudomembranous colitis) has been reported in a breastfeeding infant whose mother ingested ciprofloxacin. It is reported that lomefloxacin is excreted in the milk of lactating animals although levels are low.

LOPERAMIDE; *Imodium, Pepto Diarrhea Control, Maalox Anti-Diarrheal Caplets, Kaopectate II Caplets, Imodium Advanced, Novo-Loperamide*	L2
Uses: Antidiarrheal drug	B

AAP: Maternal medication usually compatible with breastfeeding

T½= 10.8 hours; **RID=** 0.03%; **Oral =** 0.3%; **MW=** 477

Clinical: Transfer of loperamide into breast milk and oral absorption is minimal. Thus, loperamide is probably safe to use during breastfeeding.

LORACARBEF; *Lorabid*	L2
Uses: Synthetic penicillin-like antibiotic	B

AAP: Not reviewed

T½= 1 hour; **RID=** ; **Oral =** 90%; **MW=**

Clinical: Loracarbef is a synthetic beta-lactam antibiotic. It is structurally similar to the cephalosporin family. It is used for gram negative and gram positive infections. Pediatric indications are available for infants 6 months and children to 12 years of age. No data are available on levels in breastmilk.

LORATADINE; *Claritin*	L1
Uses: Long-acting antihistamine	B

AAP: Maternal medication usually compatible with breastfeeding

T½= 8.4-28 hours; **RID=** 0.3%; **Oral =** Complete; **MW=** 383

Clinical: Loratadine is safe to use in breastfeeding. It is preferred over other antihistamines since it is non-sedating. Transfer into milk is negligible. No adverse effects are expected. Loratadine does not transfer into the CNS of adults, so it is unlikely to induce sedation even in infants. The half-life in neonates is not known although it is likely quite long. Pediatric formulations are available.

LORAZEPAM; *Ativan, Apo-Lorazepam, Novo-Lorazepam*	L3
Uses: Antianxiety, sedative drug	D

AAP: Drugs whose effect on nursing infants is unknown but may be of concern

T½= 12 hours;   **RID**= 2.9%;   **Oral** = 90%;   **MW**= 321

Clinical: Lorazepam transfer into human milk is minimal, and it is the ideal choice for use in breastfeeding since it has a shorter half-life and is not as addicting. Observe for sedation and withdrawal in the breastfed infant.

LORMETAZEPAM	L3
Uses: Hypntic sedative	D

AAP: Not reviewed

T½= 10-12 hours;   **RID**= ;   **Oral** = 80%;   **MW**= 335.2

Clinical: Levels of lormetazepam are apparently quite low in milk and breastfed infants. No untoward effects were reported. Lormetazepam is a benzodiazepine available in the UK. No free lormetazepam was found in the infants' plasma, nor were any adverse side effects noted in these infants.

LOSARTAN; *Cozaar, Hyzaar*	L3
Uses: ACE-like antihypertensive	C

AAP: Not reviewed

T½= 4-9 hours (metabolite);   **RID**= ;   **Oral** = 25-33%;   **MW**=

Clinical: Losartan is a new ACE-like antihypertensive. No data are available on its transfer to human milk. Although it penetrates the CNS significantly, its high protein binding would probably reduce its ability to enter milk. No data on transfer into human milk are available. Use with caution in mothers with premature infants.

LOVASTATIN; *Mevacor, Apo-Lovastatin*	L3
Uses: Hypocholesterolemic	X

AAP: Not reviewed

T½= 1.1-1.7;   **RID**= ;   **Oral** = 5-30%;   **MW**= 405

Clinical: Small but unpublished levels are known to be secreted into human breastmilk. Less then 5% of a dose reaches the maternal circulation due to extensive first-pass removal by the liver. The effect on the infant is unknown, but it could reduce hepatic cholesterol synthesis. There is little justification for using such a drug during lactation, but due to the extremely small maternal plasma levels, it is unlikely that the amount in breastmilk would be clinically active. Cholesterol and other products of cholesterol biosynthesis are essential components for fetal and neonatal development, and the use of cholesterol-lowering drugs would not be advisable under most circumstances in breastfeeding mothers.

LOXAPINE; *Loxitane, Loxapac, PMS-Loxapine*	L4
Uses: CNS tranquilizer	C
AAP: Not reviewed	
T½= 19 hours; **RID=** ; **Oral** = 33%; **MW=** 328	

Clinical: Loxapine produces pharmacologic effects similar to the phenothiazines and haloperidol family. The drug does not appear to have antidepressant effects and may lower the seizure threshold. It is a powerful tranquilizer and has been found to be secreted into the milk of animals, but no data are available for human milk. This is a potent tranquilizer than could produce significant sequelae in breastfeeding infants. Caution is urged.

LSD	L5
Uses: Hallucinogen	
AAP: Not reviewed	
T½= 3 hours; **RID=** ; **Oral** = Complete; **MW=** 268	

Clinical: LSD is a power hallucinogenic drug. No data are available on transfer into breastmilk. However, due to its extreme potency and its ability to pass the blood-brain-barrier, LSD is likely to penetrate milk and produce hallucinogenic effects in the infant. This drug is definitely CONTRAINDICATED. Maternal urine may be positive for LSD for 34-120 hours post ingestion.

LUBIPROSTONE; *Amitiza*	L3
Uses: Gastrointestinal agent	C
AAP: Not reviewed	
T½= 0.9-1.4 hours; **RID=** ; **Oral** = Nil; **MW=** 390.46	

Clinical: Unabsorbed orally. Plasma levels undetectable in patients. Milk levels are likely undetectable as well. Monitor baby for signs of diarrhea but this is unlikely.

LYME DISEASE; *Lyme Disease, Borrelia*	
Uses: Borrelia burgdorferi infections	
AAP: Not reviewed	

T½= ; RID= ; Oral = ; MW=

Clinical: Lyme disease is caused by infection with the spirochete, borrelia burgdorferi. This spirochete is transferred in-utero to the fetus. Antigenic material from the spirochete is found in human milk, although we do not know if it is infectious. If diagnosed postpartum or in a breastfeeding mother, the mother should be treated immediately. Although doxycycline therapy is not definitely contraindicated in breastfeeding mothers, alternates such as amoxicillin, cefuroxime, clarithromycin, or azithromycin should be preferred.

LYSINE; *Lysine, L-Lysine*	L2
Uses: Amino acid food supplement	
AAP: Not reviewed	

T½= 3.66 hours; RID= ; Oral = 83%; MW= 146

Clinical: Lysine is a naturally occurring amino acid; the average American ingests from 6-10 grams daily. Aside from its use as a supplement in patients with poor nutrition, it is most often used for the treatment of recurrent herpes simplex infections. The risk of toxicity is considered quite low in both adults and infants. Rather high doses have been studied in infants as young as 4 months, with doses from 60 to 1080 mg L-lysine per 8 ounces of milk. In one study, only 0.54% of the administered dose of lysine was secreted into milk proteins. Further, the lysine present in milk was present as protein, not free amino acid. Therefore supplementation of breastfeeding mothers with L-lysine will probably not result in significantly elevated levels of free lysine in milk.

MAGNESIUM HYDROXIDE; *Milk of Magnesia, Citro-Mag, Phillips Milk of Magnesia*	L1
Uses: Laxative, antacid	B
AAP: Not reviewed	

$T\frac{1}{2}$= ; **RID**= ; **Oral** = 15-30%; **MW**= 58

Clinical: Poorly absorbed from maternal GI tract. Only about 15-30 % of an orally ingested magnesium product is absorbed. Magnesium rapidly deposits in bone (>50%) and is significantly distributed to tissue sites.

MAGNESIUM SULFATE; *Epsom salt*	L1
Uses: Saline laxative and anticonvulsant (IV,IM)	B

AAP: Maternal medication usually compatible with breastfeeding

$T\frac{1}{2}$= <3 hours; **RID**= 0.2%; **Oral** = 4%; **MW**= 120

Clinical: Magnesium sulfate transfers to breast milk minimally, and there have been no reports of adverse effects in breastfed infants. Levels in milk seem to drop off after a few days of administration, and are not clinically relevant.

MALATHION; *Ovide, Malathion Lotion*	L3
Uses: Pediculicide, scabicide	B

AAP: Not reviewed

$T\frac{1}{2}$= 7.6 hours; **RID**= ; **Oral** = Complete; **MW**=

Clinical: Less than 10% of malathion is absorbed transcutaneously and is rapidly metabolized and excreted. While it belongs to the organophosphate family of insecticides, it is so rapidly metabolized and eliminated by humans (10 times) that it relatively nontoxic under normal conditions. Topically, it should not be used in neonates, although one case report of its used in a 7 month-old infant suggests it is relatively safe. Less than 10% of malathion is absorbed transcutaneously and is rapidly metabolized and excreted. While it belongs to the organophosphate family of insecticides, it is so rapidly metabolized and eliminated by humans (10 times) that it relatively nontoxic under normal conditions.

MANNITOL; *Osmitrol*	L3
Uses: Osmotic diuretic	C

AAP: Not reviewed

$T\frac{1}{2}$= 71-100 minutes; **RID**= ; **Oral** = 17%; **MW**= 182

Clinical: It is not known if it enters the milk compartment, but it is likely only during the first few days postpartum when the tight-junctions in the alveolar system are immature. After 48-72 hours the entry of mannitol into human milk is probably minimal. Oral absorption in infants would be minimal except early postpartum when their GI tract is relative porous. The elimination half-life is 71-100 minutes.

MAPROTILINE; *Ludiomil, Novo-Maprotilene*	L3
Uses: Antidepressant	B
AAP: Not reviewed	
T½= 27-58 hours; **RID=** 1.4%; **Oral =** 100%; **MW=** 277	
Clinical: Milk/plasma ratios varied from 1.3 to 1.5. While these levels are quite low, it is not known if they are hazardous to a breastfed infant, but caution is recommended.	

MEASLES VIRUS VACCINE, LIVE	L3
Uses: Vaccination for Measles	
AAP: Not reviewed	
T½= ; **RID=** ; **Oral =** ; **MW=**	
Clinical: Rubella, and perhaps measles and mumps virus, are undoubtedly transferred via breastmilk and have been detected in throat swabs of 56% of breastfeeding infants. Infants exposed to the attenuated viruses via breastmilk had only mild symptoms. If medically required, MMR vaccine can be administered early postpartum.	

MEBENDAZOLE; *Vermox*	L3
Uses: Anthelmintic	C
AAP: Not reviewed	
T½= 2.8-9 hours; **RID=** ; **Oral =** 2-10%; **MW=** 295	
Clinical: Considering the poor oral absorption and high protein binding, it is unlikely that mebendazole would be transmitted to the infant in clinically relevant concentrations.	

MECLIZINE; *Antivert, Bonine, Bonamine*	L3
Uses: Antiemetic, antivertigo, motion sickness	B
AAP: Not reviewed	

T½= 6 hours; **RID**= ; **Oral** = Complete; **MW**= 391

Clinical: We have no data on the transfer of meclizine into human milk. The use of meclizine while breastfeeding is probably safe, however monitoring for sedation in the infant is advised.

MEDROXYPROGESTERONE AND ESTRADIOL CYPIONATE; *Lunelle*	L3
Uses: Once-a-month birth control injection	X

AAP: Not reviewed

T½= ; **RID**= ; **Oral** = ; **MW**=

Clinical: Although small amounts of estrogens and progestins may pass into breastmilk, the effects of these hormones on an infant appear minimal. Use of estrogen containing products, particularly early postpartum, may dramatically reduce the volume of milk produced. Mothers should attempt to delay use of these products for as long as possible postpartum (at least 6-8 weeks), if at all. Because of the estrogen content and the prolonged release formula, caution is recommended in breastfeeding mothers.

MEDROXYPROGESTERONE; *Provera, Depo-Provera, Cycrin, Alti-MPA, Gen-Medroxy*	L1
Uses: Injectable progestational agent	X

AAP: Maternal medication usually compatible with breastfeeding

T½= 14.5 hours; **RID**= ; **Oral** = 0.6-10%; **MW**= 344

Clinical: Progestin-only contraceptives are generally regarded as safe, although it is best to start after 6 weeks post-partum. Studies have concluded that there are no risks of breastfed infants having growth and developmental impairmentg. However, we have many clinical reports of reduced milk supply in mothers who received progestin products. In some instances, it might be advisable to recommend treatment with oral progestin-only contraceptives postpartum rather than DMPA, so that women who experience reduced milk supply could easily withdraw from the medication without significant loss of breast milk supply. Progestins should be avoided early postnatally, and perhaps longer.

MEFLOQUINE; *Lariam*	L2
Uses: Antimalarial	C

AAP: Not reviewed

T½= 10-21 days;   **RID=** 0.1% - 0.2%;   **Oral =** 85%;   **MW=** 414

Clinical: Mefloquine is secreted in small concentrations approximating 3% of the maternal dose which is not sufficient to protect the infant from malaria. Thus far, no untoward effects have been reported but discontinue if neuropsychiatric disturbances occur.

MELATONIN	L3

Uses: Hormone

AAP: Not reviewed

T½= 30-50 minutes;   **RID=** ;   **Oral =** Complete;   **MW=** 232

Clinical: Melatonin is a normal hormone secreted by the pineal gland in the human brain. It is known to be passed into human milk and is believed responsible for entraining the newborn brain to phase shift its circadian clock to that of the mother. The effect of orally administered melatonin on newborns is unknown, but melatonin has thus far not been associated with significant untoward effects.

MELOXICAM; *Mobic*	L3

Uses: Nonsteroidal anti-inflammatory agent   C

AAP: Not reviewed

T½= 20.1 hours;   **RID=** ;   **Oral =** 89%;   **MW=** 351

Clinical: No data are available for transfer into human milk although it does transfer into rodent milk. Due to its long half-life and good bioavailability, another NSAID would probably be preferred such as ibuprofen or celecoxib (Celebrex). Observe for diarrhea.

MEMANTINE; *Namenda, Ebixa*	L3

Uses: NMDA Receptor Antagonist   B

AAP: Not reviewed

T½= 60-80 hours;   **RID=** ;   **Oral =** Complete;   **MW=** 216

Clinical: No data are availble, but due to its large volume of distribution, milk levels will probably be minimal.

MENINGOCOCCAL VACCINE; *Menomune, Menveo*	L1
Uses: Vaccine	C
AAP: Not reviewed	
T½= ; **RID=** ; **Oral =** ; **MW=**	
Clinical: Meningococcal polysaccharide vaccine is a freeze-dried preparation of group-specific antigens from Neisseria meningitidis. This vaccine is not infectious. This vaccine is useful to prevent endemic and epidemic meningitis and meningococcemia in children and young adults. There are no known contraindications for using this in breastfeeding mothers other than allergic hypersensitivity to some of the ingredients.	

MENOTROPINS; *Pergonal, Humegon, Repronex*	L3
Uses: Produces follicle growth	X
AAP: Not reviewed	
T½= 3.9 and 70.4 hours; **RID=** ; **Oral =** 0%; **MW=** 34,000	
Clinical: Menotropins is a purified preparation of gonadotropins hormones (follicle stimulating hormone (FSH) and luteinizing hormone (LH)). These hormones are large molecular weight peptides and would not likely penetrate into human milk. Further, they are unstable in the GI tract and their oral bioavailability would be minimal to zero even in an infant.	

MEPERIDINE; *Demerol, Pethidine*	L2
Uses: Narcotic analgesic	C
AAP: Maternal medication usually compatible with breastfeeding	
T½= 3.2 hours; **RID=** 1.4% - 13.9%; **Oral =** <50%; **MW=** 247	
Clinical: Meperidine is not recommended for use during breastfeeding, as its metabolite has a very long half-life, and may cause sedation and poor suckling in the breastfed infant. One time use may be okay in an older infant. Chronic or epidural use is not advised in women intending to breastfeed.	

MEPINDOLOL SULFATE	L2
Uses: Non-specific beta blocker	C
AAP: Not reviewed	
T½= 3-4 hours; **RID=** 1%; **Oral =** >95%; **MW=**	

Clinical: The RID is 1%. One study of 5 infants found no untoward effects. No drug-related side effects were noted in these 5 infants.

MEPIVACAINE; *Carbocaine, Polocaine*	L3
Uses: Local anesthetic	C
AAP: Not reviewed	
T½= 1.9-3.2 hours; **RID=** ; **Oral =** ; **MW=**	

Clinical: Mepivacaine is a long acting local anesthetic similar to bupivacaine. No data are available on the transfer of mepivacaine into human milk but bupivacaine enters milk in exceedingly low levels. Due to higher fetal levels and reported toxicities, mepivacaine is never used antenatally. For use in breastfeeding patients, bupivacaine is preferred.

MEPROBAMATE; *Equanil, Miltown, Novo-Mepro, Apo-Meprobamate*	L3
Uses: Antianxiety drug	D
AAP: Not reviewed	
T½= 6-17 hours; **RID=** ; **Oral =** Complete; **MW=** 218	

Clinical: Meprobamate is secreted into milk at levels 2-4 times that of the maternal plasma level. It could produce some sedation in a breastfeeding infant.

MERCAPTOPURINE; *Purinethol, 6-MP*	L3
Uses: Antimetabolite, immunosuppressant	D
AAP: Not reviewed	
T½= 21-90 minutes; **RID=** ; **Oral =** 50%; **MW=** 170	

Clinical: Mercaptopurine is the active metabolite of azathioprine. The transfer of the active metabolite (6-MP) into milk is quite low. However, this is a strong immunosuppressant and some caution is still recommended. Monitor the infant closely for signs of immunosuppression, leukopenia, thrombocytopenia, hepatotoxicity, and pancreatitis. The risks to the infant are probably low.

MERCURY; *Mercury*	L5
Uses: Environmental contaminate	X
AAP: Not reviewed	

T½= 70 days; **RID=** ; **Oral** = Variable; **MW=** 201

Clinical: Mercury transfers into human milk with a milk/plasma ratio that varies according to the mercury form. Concentrations of mercury in human milk are generally much higher in populations that ingest large quantities of fish. Mothers known to be contaminated with mercury should not breastfeed. Exposure to mercury of breastfed infants from maternal amalgam fillings is of minor importance compared to maternal fish consumption. The replacement of amalgam fillings should if possible be postponed until after pregnancy, and breastfeeding as the removal of amalgam fillings while breastfeeding could potentially increase the transfer of mercury to the breastfed infant and largely (this largely depends on the precautions taken by the dentist).

MEROPENEM; *Merrem*	L3
Uses: Semisynthetic carbapenem antibiotic	B

AAP: Not reviewed

T½= 1 hour; **RID=** ; **Oral** = Nil; **MW=** 437

Clinical: No data are available on its transfer into human milk but like others in this family, it is likely low. Further this agent is not orally bioavailable to any degree. Observe for diarrhea in breastfed infants.   Changes in gut flora could be expected in breastfed infants.

MESALAMINE; *Asacol, Pentasa, Rowasa, Canasa, Lialda, Salofalk, Mesasal, Quintasa*	L3
Uses: Antiinflammatory in ulcerative colitis	B

AAP: Should be given to nursing mothers with caution

T½= 5-10 hours (metabolite); **RID=** 0.1% - 8.8%; **Oral** = 20-30%; **MW=** 153

Clinical: Numerous reports suggest milk levels of 5 aminosalicylic acid are quite low, generally less than 10% of the maternal dose. However, the dose used seems to be going up and the new Lialda now has a 4.5 gm dosage form. At these doses, milk levels of 5-aminosalicylic acid and even salicylic acid could become signficiant. Watery diarrhea has been reported but this appears to be rare. Commonly used in many patients without reported complications. Observe infant for GI symptoms.

MESORIDAZINE; *Serentil*	**L4**
Uses: Phenothiazine antipsychotic	C

AAP: Drugs whose effect on nursing infants is unknown but may be of concern

T½= 24-48 hours; **RID=** ; **Oral** = Erratic; **MW=**

Clinical: Mesoridazine is a typical phenothiazine antipsychotic used for treatment of schizophrenia. No data on transfer into human milk are available. However, the use of the phenothiazine family in breastfeeding mothers is risky and may increase the risk of SIDS.

METAMIZOLE; *Dipyrone, Algosfar, Algozone, Analagin, Novalgin Melubrin, Novalgina*	**L3**
Uses: Analgesic, antipyretic	

AAP: Not reviewed

T½= 2-3 hours (4-MAA); **RID=** 1.2%; **Oral** = Complete; **MW=** 311

Clinical: Because of its known complications, such as agranulocytosis and other blood dyscrasias, metamizole is no longer recommended as an analgesic in many countries. Other safer alternatives are available such as acetaminophen and ibuprofen. However, in severe life-threatening and refractory fever, it is a suitable antipyretic. All metabolites are undetectable by 48 hours.

METAXALONE; *Skelaxin*	**L3**
Uses: Sedative, skeletal muscle relaxant	C

AAP: Not reviewed

T½= 2-3 hours; **RID=** ; **Oral** = ; **MW=** 221

Clinical: No data are available on its transfer into breastmilk. No data available for pediatric concerns. Can cause sedation, nausea, vomiting, anemia and abnormal liver function in adults.

METFORMIN; *Glucophage, Glucovance, Riomet, Gen-Metformin, Glycon*	**L1**
Uses: Oral hypoglycemic agent for diabetes	B

AAP: Not reviewed

T½= 6.2 hours (plasma); **RID=** 0.3% - 0.7%; **Oral** = 50%; **MW=** 129

Clinical: Metformin is safe to use during breastfeeding, and has been used with no untoward effects in the breastfed infant. Transfer to milk is minimal, and plasma levels are undetected in the breastfed infant. Determine if the patient is on other diabetic medications.

METHACHOLINE CHLORIDE; *Arthralgen, Mecholyl, Provocholine*	L3
Uses: Bronchoconstrictor used for diagnosis of asthma	C

AAP: Not reviewed

T½= Brief; **RID=** ; **Oral** = Low to nil; **MW**= 195

Clinical: Methacholine is poorly absorbed orally and would have minimal transport into the milk compartment. It is also unlikely to survive the GI tract. Because this is a one-time test, for asthma a brief interruption of breastfeeding for a few hours (4) would all but eliminate any risk.

METHADONE; *Dolophine, Metadon*	L3
Uses: Narcotic analgesic	C

AAP: Maternal medication usually compatible with breastfeeding

T½= 13-55 hours; **RID=** 1.9% - 6.5%; **Oral** = 50%; **MW**= 309

Clinical: Methadone has been used in many breastfeeding mothers, and is usually compatible with breastfeeding. Even high doses of methadone transfer only small amounts into human milk. Observe for sedation, withdrawal, addiction in the breastfed infant. Methadone while breastfeeding actually alleviates some of the symptoms of neonatal abstinence syndrome. In summary, the dose of methadone transferred via milk is largely dose dependent but generally averages less than 2.8% of the maternal dose. This is significantly less than the conventional cut-off value of 10% of the maternal dose corrected for weight. The Academy of Pediatrics has placed methadone in the "approved" category for breastfeeding women.

METHAMPHETAMINE; *Desoxyephedrine Desoxyn, Pervitin, Anadrex, Methedrine*	L5
Uses: CNS Stimulant	C

AAP: Advise not to breastfeed

T½= 4-13.6 hours; **RID=** ; **Oral** = 63%; **MW**= 185.7

Clinical: Breastfeeding mothers should avoid using this drug, or pump and discard milk for at least 48 hours. Methamphetamine is a strong CNS stimulant that is strongly addictive. After prolonged use it is known to induce paranoid symptoms. Breastfeeding mothers should avoid using this drug, or pump and discard milk for at least 48 hours.

METHICILLIN; *Staphcillin, Celbenin*	L3
Uses: Penicillin antibiotic	B
AAP: Not reviewed	

T½= 1-2 hours; **RID**= ; **Oral** = Poor; **MW**= 402

Clinical: No data are available on the transfer into breastmilk although it would appear to be similar to other penicillins such as dicloxicillin which has minimal concentrations in breastmilk. Observe for diarrhea.

METHIMAZOLE; *Tapazole*	L3
Uses: Antithyroid agent	D
AAP: Maternal medication usually compatible with breastfeeding	

T½= 6-13 hours; **RID**= 2.3%; **Oral** = 80-95%; **MW**= 114

Clinical: Methimazole usage during breastfeeding is probably safe. There are lots of data reporting no untoward effects to the infant for periods up to 12 months. Monitor thyroid function of the breastfed infant to be safe. In a large study of over 139 thyrotoxic lactating mothers and their infants, even at methimazole doses of 20 mg/day, no changes in infant TSH, T4 or T3 were noted in over 12 months of study. The authors conclude that both PTU and methimazole can safely be administered during lactation. However, during the first few months of therapy, monitoring of infant thyroid functioning is recommended.

METHOCARBAMOL; *Robaxisal, Robaxin*	L3
Uses: Muscle relaxant	C
AAP: Not reviewed	

T½= 0.9-1.8 hours; **RID**= ; **Oral** = Complete; **MW**= 241

Clinical: Only minimal amounts have been found in milk. No pediatric concerns but studies are limited. Observe for sedation.

METHOHEXITAL; *Brevital, Brietal*	L3
Uses: Anesthetic agent	B

AAP: Maternal medication usually compatible with breastfeeding

T½= 3.9 hours; **RID**= 2.8%; **Oral** = ; **MW**= 262

Clinical: Methohexital is an anesthetic agent (barbiturate). Milk levels are reportedly very low due to being distributed into adipose tissue within 30 minutes of dose. A brief wait of two hours or so would completely eliminate any risk.

METHOTREXATE; *Folex, Rheumatrex*	L3
Uses: Antimetabolite, anticancer, antirheumatic	X

AAP: Cytotoxic drug that may interfere with cellular metabolism of the nursing infant

T½= 8-15 hours; **RID**= 0.1%; **Oral** = 33-90%; **MW**= 454

Clinical: Methotrexate is secreted into milk in small doses, but the half life increases at high and repeated doses. The drug is believed to be retained in GI and ovarian tissue for extended periods (months). Repeated doses of greater than 50 mg (high dose), the patient should not breastfeed. One high dose only, patient may pump and discard milk for 4 days then resume breastfeeding. If a low dose is given once weekly (less than 50 mg), then the mother may pump and discard milk for 24 hrs then resume breastfeeding. If the patient must have repeated low dose treatments such as three times per week, then she should not breastfeed. Patients with poor renal function have prolonged methotrexate half-lives.

METHSCOPOLAMINE; *Pamine, Aerohist, AlleRx, Amdry-D*	L3
Uses: Anticholinergic, antispasmotic	C

AAP: Not reviewed

T½= <4 hours; **RID**= ; **Oral** = 10-25%; **MW**= 398

Clinical: Methscopolamine is a quarternary ammonium compound, which would suggest that its entry into human milk would be negligible. Further, its oral bioavailability is low as well (10-25%). Taken together, these two facts would suggest that methscopolamine is not a likely problem for a breastfeeding infant. However, we do not have data yet on this product in breastfeeding mothers. Old anectdotal data persists suggesting that anticholinergics suppress milk production. This is probably not true in my opinion. This product could probably be used with care in breastfeeding mothers while observing the infant for classical anticholinergic symptoms.

METHYLCELLULOSE	L1

Uses: Laxative

AAP: Not reviewed

T½= ; RID= ; Oral = ; MW=

Clinical: There are no data on the excretion of methylcellulose into human milk. However, it stays in the GI tract and is unabsorbed. It is safe for breastfeeding mothers.

METHYLDOPA; *Aldomet, Apo-Methyldopa, Dopamet, Nova-Medopa*	L2

Uses: Antihypertensive | B

AAP: Maternal medication usually compatible with breastfeeding

T½= 105 minutes; RID= 0.1% - 0.3%; Oral = 25-50%; MW= 211

Clinical: Methyldopa is probably safe to use during breastfeeding. The levels of methyldopa transferred into milk are minimal. One case report of gynecomastia and galactorrhea in a two-week old breastfed infant. In general, no adverse effects are reported in breastfed infants.

METHYLENE BLUE; *Dolsed, Atrosept, Prosed, Urimar-T*	L4

Uses: Diagnostic Agent | C

AAP: Not reviewed

T½= 5.25; RID= ; Oral = ; MW= 319

Clinical: No data are available on its transfer into human milk, but some should be expected. Oral absorption is considered poor. The apparent half-life in humans is approximately 5.25 hours, thus interruption of breastfeeding for 24 hours is probably advisable.

METHYLERGONOVINE; *Methergine*	L2
Uses: Vasoconstrictor, uterine stimulant	C
AAP: Not reviewed	

T½= 20-30 minutes; RID= 2%; Oral = 60%; MW= 339

Clinical: Methylergonovine may suppress prolactin in certain patients under certain conditions. However, the infrequent or single use of this medication will probably not have much affect on prolactin levels or milk production. Avoid prolonged use however.

METHYLPHENIDATE; *Ritalin, Concerta, Metadate CD, Metadate ER, Methylin, Daytrana, Focalin XR, PMS-Methylphenidate, Riphenidate*	L3
Uses: CNS stimulant, treatment of ADHD	C
AAP: Not reviewed	

T½= 1.4-4.2 hours; RID= 0.2% - 0.4%; Oral = 95%; MW= 233

Clinical: Average methylphenidate levels in milk are only 19 ug/L. The average relative infant dose was only 0.9%. In the one infant studied, plasma levels were < 1 ug/L. These levels are probably too low to be clinically relevant. No adverse effects were noted in any of the infants.

METHYLPREDNISOLONE; *Solu-Medrol, Depo-Medrol, Medrol*	L2
Uses: Corticosteroid	C
AAP: Maternal medication usually compatible with breastfeeding	

T½= 2.8 hours; RID= ; Oral = Complete; MW= 374

Clinical: Methylprednisonolone is probably safe to use during breastfeeding as long as it is taken in low-moderate doses. Do not exceed 80 mg daily. If high doses are needed, it may be advisable to pump and discard milk for 24 hours. Observe for impaired bone growth, induce gastric ulcerations, glaucoma. No adverse effects in the breastfed infant have been reported.

METOCLOPRAMIDE; *Reglan, Metozolv ODT, Apo-Metoclop, Emex, Maxeran*	L2

Uses: GI stimulant, prolactin stimulant	B

AAP: Drugs whose effect on nursing infants is unknown but may be of concern

T½= 5-6 hours; **RID=** 4.7% - 14.3%; **Oral =** 30-100%; **MW=** 300

Clinical: Metoclopramide effectively elevated plasma prolactin levels in breastfeeding patients. In those with predisposing lower levels, this increase may increase milk synthesis. In those patients with already high levels (>100 ng/mL), metoclopramide may not work. Observed for sedation and depression in mothers following prolonged therapy. No reported pediatric adverse outcomes have been reported via milk. The drug is used commonly in pediatrics. Two recent cases of serotonin-like reactions (agitation, dysarthria, diaphoresis and extrapyramidal movement disorder) have been reported when metoclopramide was used in patients receiving sertraline or venlafaxine. The FDA has recently warned of symptoms of tardive dyskinesia after 3 months of exposure.

METOPROLOL; *Toprol-XL, Lopressor, Apo-Metoprolol, Betaloc, Novo-Metoprol*	L3

Uses: Antihypertensive, beta blocker	C

AAP: Maternal medication usually compatible with breastfeeding

T½= 3-7 hours; **RID=** 1.4%; **Oral =** 40-50%; **MW=** 267

Clinical: Metoprolol milk levels are low. Metoprolol is probably safe to use during breastfeeding. Although no pediatric adverse effects have been seen in several studies, observe for hypotension, weakness, and bradycardia in the breastfed infant. Although the milk/plasma ratios for this drug are in general high, the maternal plasma levels are quite small so the absolute amount transferred to the infant are quite small. Although these levels are probably too low to be clinically relevant, clinicians should use metoprolol under close supervision.

METRONIDAZOLE TOPICAL GEL; *MetroGel Topical, Metro-Gel*	L3

Uses: Topical antibacterial	B

AAP: Not reviewed

T½= 8.5 hours; **RID=** ; **Oral =** Complete; **MW=** 171

Clinical: Applied topically, metronidazole transfers minimally into milk, and is probably safe to use during breastfeeding. There have been no reports of adverse effects.

METRONIDAZOLE VAGINAL GEL; *MetroGel Vaginal*	L2
Uses: Antibiotic	B

AAP: Drugs whose effect on nursing infants is unknown but may be of concern

T½= 8.5 hours; **RID=** ; **Oral** = Complete; **MW=** 171

Clinical: Both topical and vaginal preparations of metronidazole contain only 0.75% metronidazole. Milk levels following intravaginal use would probably be exceedingly low. Metronidazole is used in preterm neonates, infants, and children. No adverse pediatric effects in several studies.

METRONIDAZOLE; *Flagyl, Metizol, Trikacide, Protostat, Noritate, Apo-Metronidazole, NeoMetric, Novo-Nidazol*	L2
Uses: Antibiotic, amebicide	B

AAP: Drugs whose effect on nursing infants is unknown but may be of concern

T½= 8.5 hours; **RID=** 12.6% - 13.5%; **Oral** = 100%; **MW=** 171

Clinical: Transfer of metronidazole to breast milk is significant. However it is safe to use during breastfeeding, since it is commonly used in premature infants at much higher therapeutic doses. There have been no reports of adverse effects in breastfed infants.

METYRAPONE; *Metopirone*	L2
Uses: Diagnostic agent, radiopharmaceutical imaging	C

AAP: Not reviewed

T½= ; **RID=** 0.06%; **Oral** = Complete; **MW=** 226

Clinical: Metyrapone is a diagnostic drug for diagnosis and treatment of adrenocortical hyperfunction. The authors of a case report suggest that maternal metyrapone use during breastfeeding is unlikely to be a significant risk to an infant.

MEXILETINE HCL; *Mexitil, Novo-Mexiletine*	L2
Uses: Antiarrhythmic	C

AAP: Maternal medication usually compatible with breastfeeding

T½= 9.2 hours; **RID=** 1.4% - 1.6%; **Oral =** 90%; **MW=** 179

Clinical: Mexiletine is an antiarrhythmic agent with activity similar to lidocaine. Milk levels are low. It is unlikely that exposure would lead to untoward side effects in a breastfeeding infant.

MICONAZOLE; *Monistat IV, Monistat 3, 7, Oravig, Micatin, Monistat*	L2
Uses: Antifungal for candidiasis	C

AAP: Not reviewed

T½= 20-25 hours; **RID=** ; **Oral =** 25-30%; **MW=** 416

Clinical: Intravaginal and topical administration of miconazole have very low systemic absorption, and so it is highly unlikely to transfer to human milk. Oral and intravenous administration may likely transfer to milk, however it is still probably safe to use during breastfeeding. Miconazole is commonly used in infants therapeutically.

MIDAZOLAM; *Versed*	L2
Uses: Short acting benzodiazepine sedative, hypnotic	D

AAP: Drugs whose effect on nursing infants is unknown but may be of concern

T½= 2-5 hours; **RID=** 0.6%; **Oral =** 27-44%; **MW=** 326

Clinical: Midazolam is rapidly redistributed from the plasma compartment to other tissue compartments and therefore milk levels will be low. Breastfeeding may be restarted after 4 hours.

MIDODRINE; *ProAmatine, Amatine*	L3
Uses: Vasopressor / antihypotensive agent	C

AAP: Not reviewed

T½= 3-4 hours (metabolite); **RID=** ; **Oral =** 93%; **MW=** 290

Clinical: No data are available on its transfer to human milk, but some should be expected. This product is small in molecular weight, belongs to the phenylethylamine family, is lipophilic, and is likely to penetrate milk as do the other members of this family. Some caution is recommended. Observe infant for hypertension, insomnia, and excitement.

MIFEPRISTONE; *Mifeprex, Mifegyn, Pencroftonum*	L3
Uses: Antiprogestational agent	X
AAP: Not reviewed	

T½= 18 hours; **RID**= ; **Oral** = 69%; **MW**= 426

Clinical: Mifepristone is used to terminate pregnancies. No data are available on its transfer into human milk, but small levels probably do enter the milk compartment. No studies are available in humans. It has interestingly been used in monkeys to increase milk production.

MIGLITOL; *Glyset, Diastabol*	L2
Uses: Anti diabetic agent	B
AAP: Not reviewed	

T½= 2 hours; **RID**= 0.4%; **Oral** = Variable; **MW**= 207

Clinical: The manufacturer reports that milk levels are very small. The manufacturer reports that milk levels are very small. Total excretion into milk accounted for 0.02% of a 100 mg maternal dose. The estimated exposure to a nursing infant is approximately 0.4% of the maternal dose.

MILK THISTLE; *Holy Thistle, Lady Thistle, Marian Thistle, Silybum, Silymarin*	L3
Uses: Hepatoprotectant	
AAP: Not reviewed	

T½= ; **RID**= ; **Oral** = 23-47%; **MW**= 482

Clinical: No data are available concerning Silymarin transfer to human milk but some probably transfers. However, it is rather devoid of reported toxicity with only brief GI intolerance and mild allergic reactions for adults. No pediatric concerns have been reported via milk.

MINOCYCLINE;   *Minocin, Dynacin, Arestin, Novo-Minocycline*   L2

Uses: Tetracycline antibiotic   D

AAP: Not reviewed

T½= 15-20 hours; **RID=** 0.2% - 1.4%; **Oral =** 90-100%; **MW=** 457

Clinical: Short-term usage (<3 weeks) is probably okay, however not recommended as there are many other antibiotics out there that do not stain the teeth or impair growth. Prolonged usage is ill-advised. There is little risk of permanent dental staining with only a brief exposure (three weeks).

MINOXIDIL;   *Loniten, Minodyl, Rogaine, Apo-Gain, Minox*   L2

Uses: Antihypertensive   C

AAP: Maternal medication usually compatible with breastfeeding

T½= 3.5-4.2 hours; **RID=** 9.1%; **Oral =** 90-95%; **MW=** 209

Clinical: Long-term exposure of breastfeeding infants in women ingesting oral minoxidil may not be advisable. However, in those using topical minoxidil, the limited absorption via skin would minimize systemic levels and significantly reduce risk of transfer to infant via breastmilk. It is unlikely that the amount absorbed via topical application would produce clinically relevant concentrations in breastmilk.

MIRTAZAPINE;   *Remeron*   L3

Uses: Antidepressant   C

AAP: Not reviewed

T½= 20-40 hours; **RID=** 1.6% - 6.3%; **Oral =** 50%; **MW=** 265

Clinical: Milk levels appear quite small. But this is an antidepressant with strong sedative properties. Observe infant for sedation. RID 1.6-6.3%. Alternatives: sertraline, venlafaxine, or paroxetine

MISOPROSTOL;   *Cytotec*   L3

Uses: Prostaglandin hormone, gastric protectant   X

AAP: Not reviewed

T½= 20-40 minutes; **RID=** ; **Oral =** Complete; **MW=** 383

Clinical: This cytokine while present in milk is quite low as indicated by a milk/plasma ratio of only 0.05. andRecommendation is to take the med. immediately after a feed then wait 4 hrs to start next feed. Observe infant for diarrhea and abdominal cramping (GI effects unlikely).

MITOXANTRONE; *Novantrone*	L5
Uses: Immunosuppressant for MS	D
AAP: Not reviewed	
T½= 23-215 hours; **RID=** ; **Oral** = Poor; **MW=** 517	
Clinical: Mitoxantrone is an antineoplastic agent used in the treatment of relapsing multiple sclerosis. It has a large volume of distribution leading to prolonged tissue, plasma, and milk levels. As this is a DNA-reactive agent, and it has a huge volume of distribution leading to prolonged tissue, plasma, and milk levels, mothers should be strongly advised to not breastfeed following its use.	

MIVACURIUM; *Mivacron, Mivacrom*	L2
Uses: Neuromuscular blocking agent	C
AAP: Not reviewed	
T½= <30 minutes; **RID=** ; **Oral** = Poor; **MW=**	
Clinical: No data are available on its transfer to breastmilk. However, it has an exceedingly short plasma half-life (< 30 minutes) and probably poor to no oral absorption. It is very unlikely that it would be absorbed by a breastfeeding infant.	

MMR VACCINE; *MMR Vaccine, Measles - Mumps - Rubella*	L2
Uses: Live attenuated triple virus vaccine	C
AAP: Not reviewed	
T½= ; **RID=** ; **Oral** = ; **MW=**	
Clinical: Rubella, and perhaps measles and mumps virus, are transferred via breastmilk and have been detected in throat swabs of 56% of breastfeeding infants. Infants exposed to the attenuated viruses via breastmilk had only mild symptoms. If medically required, MMR vaccine can be administered early postpartum.	

MOCLOBEMIDE; *Apo-Moclobemide, Manerix*	L3
Uses: MAO inhibitor, antidepressant.	
AAP: Not reviewed	

T½= 1-2.2 hours; **RID=** 3.4%; **Oral** = 80%; **MW=** 269

Clinical: Unlike older MAO inhibitors, moclobemide is a selective and reversible inhibitor of MAO-A and thus is not plagued with the dangerous side effects of the older MAO inhibitor families. In one study the average milk concentration throughout the 12 hour period was 0.97 mg/L hour. The minimal levels of moclobemide found in milk are unlikely to produce untoward effects according to the authors.

MODAFINIL; *Provigil, Alertec*	L4
Uses: Wakefulness-promoting agent	C
AAP: Not reviewed	

T½= 15 hours; **RID=** ; **Oral** = Complete; **MW=** 273

Clinical: Modafinil is a wakefulness-promoting agent used for the treatment of narcolepsy. Although its pharmacologic results are similar to amphetamines and methylphenidate (Ritalin), its method of action is unknown. No data are available on its transfer into human milk. Some caution is recommended as it is small in molecular weight and very lipid soluble, both characteristics which may ultimately lead to higher milk levels. In addition, it apparently stimulates dopamine levels. Compounds that stimulate dopamine levels in brain often reduce prolactin secretion. Milk production may suffer, but this is only theoretical.

MOMETASONE FUROATE + FORMOTEROL FUMATE; *Dulera*	L3
Uses: Corticosteroid + long acting beta 2 adrenergic agonist	C
AAP: Not reviewed	

T½= ; **RID=** ; **Oral** = ; **MW=**

MOMETASONE; *Elocon, Nasonex*	L3
Uses: Corticosteroid	C
AAP: Not reviewed	

T½= ; **RID=** ; **Oral** = ; **MW=**

Clinical: Mometasone is a corticosteroid primarily intended for intranasal and topical use. It is considered a medium-potency steroid, similar to betamethasone and triamcinolone. Following topical application to the skin, less than 0.7% is systemically absorbed over an 8 hour period. It is extremely unlikely mometasone would be excreted into human milk in clinically relevant levels following topical or intranasal administration.

MONOETHANOLAMINE OLEATE; *Ethamolin*	L3

Uses: Sclerosing Agent

AAP: Not reviewed

T½= ;   RID= ;   Oral = ;   MW= 344

Clinical: Monoethanolamine is a sclerosing agent to treat varicose veins. There are no data on its transfer to human milk. There are no studies done in nursing women. Pump and discard milk for 4 hours.

MONTELUKAST SODIUM; *Singulair*	L3
Uses: Antiasthmatic agent	B

AAP: Advise not to breastfeed

T½= 2.7-5.5 hours;   RID= ;   Oral = 64%;   MW= 608

Clinical: Montelukast is a leukotriene receptor inhibitor and is used as an adjunct in the treatment of asthma. The manufacturer reports that montelukast is secreted into animal milk, but no data on human milk is available. This product is cleared for use in children aged 6 and above. This product does not enter the CNS nor many other tissues. Although the milk levels in humans are unreported, they are probably quite low.

MORPHINE; *Duramorph, Infumorph, Embeda, Epimorph, Morphitec, M.O.S. MS Contin, Statex*	L3
Uses: Narcotic analgesic	C

AAP: Maternal medication usually compatible with breastfeeding

T½= 1.5-2 hours;   RID= 9.1%;   Oral = 26%;   MW= 285

Clinical: Morphine is the preferred opiae to use while breastfeeding due to its poor oral bioavailability. Do not use high doses for prolonged periods of time. Observe for sedation and constipation in the breastfed infant. Infants under 1 month of age have a prolonged elimination T ½ and decreased clearance of morphine compared to older infants.

MOXIFLOXACIN; *Avelox, Vigamox*	L2
Uses: Fluoroquinolone antibiotic	C
AAP: Not reviewed	
T½= 9-16 hours; **RID=** ; **Oral** = 90%; **MW=** 437	

Clinical: Moxifloxacin is a quinolone antibiotic for use orally, intravenously, and in the eye. It is a new-generation fluoroquinolone which exhibits improved activity against Strep. pneumonia and other species. No data are available on its transfer into human milk so until we have data, one should opt for using ofloxacin or levofloxacin for which published data is available.

MUMPS VIRUS VACCINE, LIVE	L1
Uses: Vaccination for Mumps	X
AAP: Not reviewed	
T½= ; **RID=** ; **Oral** = ; **MW=**	

Clinical: MMR vaccine is a mixture of live, attenuated viruses from measles, mumps, and rubella strains. It is usually administered to children at 12-15 months of age. NEVER administer to a pregnant woman. Rubella, and perhaps measles and mumps virus, are undoubtedly transferred via breastmilk and have been detected in throat swabs of 56% of breastfeeding infants. Infants exposed to the attenuated viruses via breastmilk had only mild symptoms. If medically required, MMR vaccine can be administered early postpartum.

MUPIROCIN OINTMENT; *Bactroban*	L1
Uses: Antibacterial ointment	B
AAP: Not reviewed	
T½= 17-36 minutes; **RID=** ; **Oral** = Complete; **MW=** 501	

Clinical: Mupirocin is a topical antibiotic used for impetigo, and other bacteria, particularly staphlococcus aureus. Mupirocin is only minimally absorbed following topical application. In one study, less than 0.3% of a topical dose was absorbed after 24 hours. Most remained adsorbed to the corneum layer of the skin. The drug is absorbed orally, but it is so rapidly metabolized that systemic levels are not sustained. It is quite safe for breastfeeding mothers.

MYCOPHENOLATE; *CellCept*	L4
Uses: Immunosuppressive agent	C

AAP: Not reviewed

T½= 17.9 hours; **RID**= ; **Oral** = 94% (parent); **MW**= 433

Clinical: Mycophenolate is an immunosuppressive agent used to prevent rejection of allogenic transplants. It is well absorbed and rapidly metabolized to MPA, the active metabolite. No data are available on its transfer into human milk. Until we have data on human breast milk levels this agent should be considered moderately hazardous.

NABUMETONE; *Relafen*	L3
Uses: Antiinflammatory agent for arthritic pain	C

AAP: Not reviewed

T½= 22-30 hours; **RID**= ; **Oral** = 38%; **MW**= 228

Clinical: It is not known if the metabolite (6MNA) is secreted in human milk. It is known to be secreted into animal milk and has a very long half-life. NSAIDS are not generally recommended in nursing mothers, except ibuprofen. Alternative: Ibuprofen.

NADOLOL; *Corgard, Syn-Nadolol, Novo-Nadolol*	L4
Uses: Antihypertensive, antianginal, beta blocker	C

AAP: Maternal medication usually compatible with breastfeeding

T½= 20-24 hours; **RID**= 4.4% - 6.9%; **Oral** = 20-40%; **MW**= 309

Clinical: Nadolol is not a preferred beta blocker due to its long half-life of 24 hours and since it tends to concentrate in the milk at levels higher than maternal plasma levels. Nadolol also transfers more easily into breast milk than other beta blockers. Suitable alternatives are metoprolol and propranolol.

NAFCILLIN; *Unipen, Nafcil*	L1
Uses: Penicillin antibiotic	B

AAP: Not reviewed

T½= 0.5-1.5 hours; **RID**= ; **Oral** = 50%; **MW**= 436

Clinical: Due to poor oral absorption, nafcillin should have little to no effect on the infant if excreted into milk. We have no data on the transfer of nafcillin into milk. Nafcillin usage during breastfeeding is probably safe. Observe for diarrhea as a side effect in the infant. Commonly used in infants with no problems.

NALBUPHINE; *Nubain*	L2
Uses: Analgesic	B

AAP: Not reviewed

T½= 5 hours; RID= 0.6%; Oral = 16%; MW= 357

Clinical: Nalbuphine is a potent narcotic analgesic similar in potency to morphine. In several studies, milk levels are exceedingly low, or less than 0.6% of the maternal dose. No complications were reported in 38 mothers-infants studied.

NALIDIXIC ACID; *NegGram*	L3
Uses: Urinary anti-infective	B

AAP: Maternal medication usually compatible with breastfeeding

T½= 1-2.5 hours; RID= 0.4% - 5.2%; Oral = 60%; MW= 232

Clinical: Nalidixic is an old fluoroquinolone and newer alternatives are preferred such as ofloxacin, ciprofloxacin or levofloxacin. Hemolytic anemia has been reported in one infant whose mother received 1 gm nalidixic acid 4 times daily. Use with extreme caution. A number of new and less toxic choices (ofloxacin) should preclude the use of this compound. Another study suggest milk levels are low, but this product should never be used today.

NALOXONE; *Narcan*	L3
Uses: Narcotic antagonist	C

AAP: Not reviewed

T½= 64 minutes; RID= ; Oral = Nil; MW= 399

Clinical: Naloxone is a narcotic antagonist that blocks the effect of many opiates. It is commonly used for the treatment of opiate overdose. Naloxone is poorly absorbed orally and plasma levels in adults are undetectable (<0.05ng/mL) two hours after oral doses. Side effects are minimal except in narcotic-addicted patients. The AAP has advised that naloxone should not be administered (directly) to infants of narcotic-dependent mothers. Its use in breastfeeding mothers would be unlikely to cause problems as its milk levels would likely be low and its oral absorption is minimal to nil.

NALTREXONE; *ReVia*	L1
Uses: Narcotic antagonist	C
AAP: Not reviewed	
$T\frac{1}{2}$= 4-13 hours; **RID**= 1.4%; **Oral** = 96%; **MW**= 341	

Clinical: Although the patient data is limited, Naltrexone levels in milk appear to be very low and virtually none is detectable in the infant's plasma compartment. The risks are probably minimal.

NAPROXEN; *Anaprox, Naprosyn, Aleve, Apo-Naproxen, Naxen*	L3
Uses: NSAID, analgesic for arthritis	C
AAP: Maternal medication usually compatible with breastfeeding	
$T\frac{1}{2}$= 12-15 hours; **RID**= 3.3%; **Oral** = 74-99%; **MW**= 230	

Clinical: The amount of naproxen transferred via milk is minimal but caution in nursing mothers should be used because of its long half-life and its effect on infant cardiovascular system, kidneys, and GI tract. However, its short term use postpartum or infrequent or occasional use would not necessarily be incompatible with breastfeeding.

NARATRIPTAN; *Amerge*	L3
Uses: Migraine headaches	C
AAP: Not reviewed	
$T\frac{1}{2}$= 6 hours; **RID**= ; **Oral** = 70%; **MW**= 372	

Clinical: No data are currently available on its transfer into human milk although the manufacturer suggests it penetrates the milk of rodents. A similar medication, sumatriptan, has been studied in breastfeeding mothers and produces minimal milk levels. Alternative: sumatriptan.

NATALIZUMAB; *Tysabri*	L3
Uses: Treatment of multiple sclerosis	C

AAP: Not reviewed

T½= 11 days; **RID=** ; **Oral** = Nil; **MW=** 149,000

Clinical: Natalizumab is a recombinant humanized IgG monoclonal antibody used to suppress immunity in patients with multiple sclerosis. Because it is a large molecular IgG, its transfer into milk is probably negligible, but as yet, we do not have data on its transfer to human milk. When small amounts of this product are added to vast quantities of IgG in the plasma, only a small percentage of natalizumab would ever be available for transport into milk. It is rather unlikely this product would be detrimental to a breastfeeding infant, but we do not know this for sure at this time.

NEBIVOLOL; *Bystolic, Nebilet, Nebicard, Nubeta, Nodon*	L3
Uses: Beta-blocker	C

AAP: Not reviewed

T½= 10-12 hours; **RID=** ; **Oral** = 12-96%; **MW=** 442

Clinical: Kinetics suggest this drug will probably have minimal milk levels, but this is as yet unknown. Some caution is recommended until more is known. Observe for sedation, tiredness, bradycardia, jitteriness. Neonatal hypoglycemia have been reported with maternal use of beta blockers.

NEDOCROMIL SODIUM; *Tilade, Mireze*	L2
Uses: Inhaled anti-inflammatory for asthmatics	B

AAP: Not reviewed

T½= 3.3 hours; **RID=** ; **Oral** = 8-17%; **MW=** 371

Clinical: Nedocromil is believed to stabilize mast cells and prevent release of bronchoconstrictors in the lung following exposure to allergens. The systemic effects are minimal due to reduced plasma levels. Systemic absorption averages less than 8-17% of the total dose even after continued dosing, which is quite low. The poor oral bioavailability of this product and the reduced side effect profile of this family of drugs suggest that it is unlikely to produce untoward effects in a nursing infant.

NEFAZODONE HCL; *Serzone*	L4
Uses: Antidepressant	C

AAP: Not reviewed

T½= 1-4 hours; **RID=** 1.2%; **Oral** = 20%; **MW=** 507

Clinical: This medication should probably not be used in breastfeeding mothers with young infants, premature infants, infants subject to apnea, or other weakened infants. Drowsiness, lethargy, failure to thrive and poor temperature control have been reported in one infant. This medication should probably not be used in breastfeeding mothers with young infants, premature infants, infants subject to apnea, or other weakened infants.

NETILMICIN; *Netromycin*	L3
Uses: Aminoglycoside antibiotic	D

AAP: Not reviewed

T½= 2-2.5 hours; **RID=** ; **Oral** = Negligible; **MW=** 476

Clinical: Netilmicin is a typical aminoglycoside antibiotic (see gentamicin). Poor oral absorption limits its use to IM and IV administration although some studies suggest significant oral absorption in infancy. Only small levels are believed to be secreted into human milk although no reports exist. See gentamicin.

NEUROMUSCULAR BLOCKING AGENTS; *Anectine, Mivacron, Tracrium, Nuromax, Pavulon, Arduan, Raplon, Zemuron, Norcuron*	L3
Uses: Muscle Relaxants for surgery	C

AAP: Not reviewed

T½= Variable; **RID=** ; **Oral** = Nil; **MW=** Large

Clinical: It is not known if any of these agents penetrate into human milk, but it is very unlikely. First they are large in molecular weight, have highly polar structures, and they are virtually excluded from most cells. Oral bioavailability is not reported, but it is likely small to nil. A brief waiting period (few hours) after surgery will eliminate most risks associated with the use of these products.

NEVIRAPINE; *Viramune*	L3
Uses: Antiretroviral agent used in HIV infections.	B

AAP: Not reviewed

T½= 25-30 hours;   **RID=** 17.8%;   **Oral** = 90%;   **MW=** 266

Clinical: Nevirapine transfers significantly into human milk and the infant. Thus infant serum levels derived following ingestion of breast milk average about 40 times higher than the IC50 for HIV even though they are only 10% of the maternal serum levels (9534 vs. 971 ng/mL). Thus far, no untoward effects have been noted in the few infants studied. It is therefore apparent, that nevirapine use by the mother might significantly reduce symptoms of infection in the infant.

NICARDIPINE; *Cardene*	L2
Uses: Antihypertensive, calcium channel blocker	C

AAP: Not reviewed

T½= 6-10 hours;   **RID=** 0.07%;   **Oral** = 35%;   **MW=** 480

Clinical: Levels in milk are extremely low, protein binding is high, and the oral bioavailability is low. It is unlikely this calcium channel blocker will produce high enough levels in milk to cause problems in a breastfeeding infant.

NICOTINE PATCHES, GUM, INHALER; *Habitrol, NicoDerm, Nicotrol, ProStep, Habitrol, Nicoderm, Nicorette, Prostep*	L2
Uses: Nicotine withdrawal systems	X

AAP: Not reviewed

T½= 2.0 hours (non-patch);   **RID=** ;   **Oral** = 30%;   **MW=** 162

Clinical: Nicotine patches are much safer to the breastfed infant than continuation of smoking during breastfeeding. The levels of nicotine in the plasma are much higher from smoking than from nicotine patches. Levels in breast milk are low, and should not cause any adverse effects. Nicotine patches are recommended for smoking cessation in breastfeeding mothers. Therefore, the risk of using nicotine patches while breastfeeding is much less than the risk of formula feeding. Mothers should be advised to limit smoking as much as possible and to smoke only after they have fed their infant, or to switch to the use of nicotine patches.

NICOTINIC ACID; *Nicobid, Nicolar, Niacels, Niacin, Nicotinamide, Niaspan*	L3
Uses: Vitamin B-3	A

AAP: Not reviewed

T½= 45 minutes; **RID=** ; **Oral =** Complete; **MW=** 123

Clinical: Lower doses are probably fine for breastfeeding mothers. However, large doses used to treat hypercholesterolemia should be avoided in breastfeeding mothers until we know more about the transfer of this drug into human milk.

NIFEDIPINE; *Adalat, Procardia, Apo-Nifed, Novo-Nifedin, Nu-Nifed*	L2
Uses: Antihypertensive calcium channel blocker	C

AAP: Maternal medication usually compatible with breastfeeding

T½= 1.8-7 hours; **RID=** 2.3% - 3.4%; **Oral =** 50%; **MW=** 346

Clinical: Transfer of nifedipine into breast milk is low, and it is probably safe to use during breastfeeding. No adverse effects have been reported in breastfed infants. Nifedipine is useful for treating nipple vasospasms. Nifedipine has been found clinically useful for nipple vasospasm. Because of the similarity to Raynaud's Phenomenon, sustained release formulations providing 30-60 mg per day are suggested.

NIMODIPINE; *Nimotop*	L2
Uses: Antihypertensive, calcium channel	C

AAP: Not reviewed

T½= 9 hours; **RID=** 0.04%; **Oral =** 13%; **MW=** 418

Clinical: Nimodipine is a calcium channel blocker although it is primarily used in preventing cerebral artery spasm and improving cerebral blood flow. The relative infant dose is quite low as are risks for the infant.

NISOLDIPINE; *Sular*	L3
Uses: Antihypertensive	C

AAP: Not reviewed

T½= 7-12 hours; **RID=** ; **Oral =** 5%; **MW=** 388

Clinical: Nisoldipine is a typical calcium channel blocker antihypertensive.   No data are available on its transfer into human milk. For alternatives see nifedipine and verapamil. Due to its poor oral bioavailability, presence of lipids which reduce its absorption, and high protein binding, it is unlikely to penetrate milk and be absorbed by the infant (undocumented).

NITAZOXANIDE; *Alinia*	L3
Uses: Antibiotic for parasitic infections	B

AAP: Not reviewed

T½= 1-1.6 hours; RID= ; Oral = Good; MW= 307

Clinical: This product is a replacement for metronidazole, although it has few advantages. Fortunately metronidazole, just like nitazoxanide has very few side effects. This is probably a suitable choice for breastfeeding women as it is also cleared for children 1 year and older. It is a suitable alternative for metronidazole in many infections including Giardia lamblia and Cryptosporidium parvum. Once absorbed it is rapidly converted to the active metabolite tizoxanide. No data are available on its transfer to human milk.

NITRAZEPAM; *Mogadon, Nitrazadon*	L2
Uses: Sedative, hypnotic	D

AAP: Not reviewed

T½= 30 hours; RID= 2.9%; Oral = 53-94%; MW= 281

Clinical: Nitrazepam is a typical benzodiazepine (Valium family) used as a sedative. In a study of 9 women who received 5 mg nitrazepam at night, the concentration in milk increased over a period of 5 days from 30 nmol/L to 48 nmol/L over 5 days. The mean milk/plasma ratio after 7 hours was 0.27 in 32 paired samples and did not vary from day 1 to day 5. The mean concentration of nitrazepam in milk was 13 µg/L and the Cmax was 0.20 µg/L. Nitrazepam levels in a 6 day old infant were below the limits of detection. No adverse effects were noted in the infants breastfed for 5 days.

NITRENDIPINE; *Baypress*	L2
Uses: Calcium channel blocker, antihypertensive	C

AAP: Not reviewed

T½= 8-11 hours; RID= ; Oral = 16-20%; MW= 360

Clinical: Nitrendipine is a typical calcium channel antihypertensive. In a group of 3 breastfeeding mothers who received 20 mg/d for 5 days, nitrendipine was excreted in breast milk at peak concentrations ranging from 4.3 to 6.5 µg/L 1-2 h after acute dosing while its inactive pyridine metabolite ranged from 6.9 to 11.9 µg/L. After 5 days of dosing, the Cmax remained in the same range and the breast milk/plasma ratio for nitrendipine was 0.2 to 0.5. On the fourth day of continuous dosing, average concentrations of nitrendipine from 24-h collections of the milk were 1.1 to 3.8 µg/L. Thus, nitrendipine and its metabolite are excreted in very low concentrations in human breast milk. Based on a maternal dose of 20 mg daily, a newborn infant would ingest an average of 1.7 µg/d of nitrendipine, or a relative dose of 0.095%.

NITROFURANTOIN; *Furadantin, Macrodantin, Furan, Macrobid, Apo-Nitrofurantoin, Nephronex*	L2
Uses: Urinary antibiotic	B
AAP: Maternal medication usually compatible with breastfeeding	
T½= 20-58 minutes; **RID**= 6.8%; **Oral** = 94%; **MW**= 238	

Clinical: Nitrofurantoin usage during breastfeeding is probably safe. Minimal levels are secreted into breast milk. Use with caution in infants with G6PD or in infants less than 1 month of age with hyperbilirubinemia.

NITROGLYCERIN, NITRATES, NITRITES; *Nitrostat, Nitrolingual, Nitrogard, Amyl Nitrite, Nitrong, Nitro-Bid, Nitroglyn, Minitran, Nitro-Dur, Nitrong SR, Nitrol, Transderm-Nitro, Nitro-Dur*	L4
Uses: Vasodilator	C
AAP: Not reviewed	
T½= 1-4 minutes; **RID**= ; **Oral** = Complete; **MW**= 227	

Clinical: Nitroglycerin is a rapid and short acting vasodilator used in angina and other cardiovascular problems including congestive heart failure. Nitroglycerin, as well as numerous other formulations (amyl nitrate, isosorbide dinitrate, etc.) all work by release of the nitrite and nitrate molecule. Two studies suggest that while nitrates/nitrites are well absorbed orally in the mother (approx. 50%), little seems to be transported to human milk. Breastfeed with caution at higher doses and with prolonged exposure. Observe the infant for methemoglobinemia.

NITROPRUSSIDE; *Nitropress, Nipride*	L4
Uses: Hypotensive agent	C

AAP: Not reviewed

T½= 3-4 minutes; **RID=** ; **Oral** = Poor; **MW=**

Clinical: Nitroprusside is a rapid acting hypotensive agent of short duration (1-10 minutes). Besides rapid hypotension, nitroprusside is converted metabolically to cyanogen (cyanide radical) which is potentially toxic. No data are available on transfer of nitroprusside nor thiocyanate into human milk. The half-life of the thiocyanate metabolite is approximately 3 days. Because the thiocyanate metabolite is orally bioavailable, some caution is advised if the mother has received nitroprusside for more than 24 hours.

NITROUS OXIDE	L3
Uses: Anesthetic gas	C

AAP: Not reviewed

T½= <3 minutes; **RID=** ; **Oral** = Poor; **MW=** 44

Clinical: Nitrous oxide is a weak anesthetic gas. It provides good analgesia and a weak anesthesia. It is rapidly eliminated from the body due to rapid exchange with nitrogen via the pulmonary alveoli (within minutes). A rapid recovery generally occurs in 3-5 minutes. Due to poor lipid solubility, uptake by adipose tissue is relatively poor, and only insignificant traces of nitrous oxide circulate in blood after discontinuing inhalation of the gas. No data exists on the entry of nitrous oxide into human milk. Ingestion of nitrous oxide orally via milk is unlikely. Chronic exposure may lead to elevated risks of fetal malformations, abortions, and bone marrow toxicity (particular in dental care workers).

NIZATIDINE; *Axid, Apo-Nizatidine*	L2
Uses: Reduces gastric acid secretion	B

AAP: Not reviewed

T½= 1.5 hours; **RID=** 0.5%; **Oral** = 94%; **MW=** 331

Clinical: Nizatidine is an antisecretory, histamine-2 antagonist that reduces stomach acid secretion. In one study of 5 lactating women using a dose of 150 mg, milk levels of nizatidine were directly proportional to circulating maternal serum levels, yet were very low. Over a 12 hour period 96 µg (less than 0.5% of dose) was secreted into the milk. No effects on infant have been reported.

NORELGESTROMIN + ETHINYL ESTRADIOL; *Ortho Evra*	L3
Uses: Patch combination contraceptive	X

AAP: Not reviewed

T½= ; **RID=** ; **Oral =** ; **MW=**

Clinical: Ortho Evra is a new combination progestin and estrogen-containing patch. It delivers approximately 150 µg/day norelgestromin and 20 µg/d ethinyl estradiol to the plasma compartment of the female. Small amounts of estrogens and progestins are known to pass into milk, but long-term follow-up of children whose mothers used combination hormonal contraceptives while breastfeeding has shown no deleterious effects on infants. Estrogen-containing contraceptives may interfere with milk production by decreasing the quantity and quality of milk production.

NORETHINDRONE AND ETHINYL ESTRADIOL; *Femhrt*	L3
Uses: Estrogen/progestin for treatment of menopausal symptoms	X

AAP: Not reviewed

T½= ; **RID=** ; **Oral =** ; **MW=**

Clinical: Estrogens are known to suppress milk production in some mothers. Although this is low dose estradiol (5 ug/d), it still may suppress milk production. Transfer of these agents to infant via milk is negligible and is of no consequence.

NORETHINDRONE; *Aygestin, Norlutate, Micronor, NOR-Q.D.*	L1
Uses: Progestin for oral contraceptives	X

AAP: Not reviewed

T½= 4-13 hours; **RID=** ; **Oral =** 60%; **MW=** 298

Clinical: This product is generally consided ideal for breastfeeding mothers. But some mothers still are quite sensitive to progestins and may suffer a loss of milk synthesis. Always warn mothers that any kind of birth control pill may suppress their milk supply, be they progestin-only, and certainly estrogen-contraining products.

NORETHYNODREL; *Enovid*	L2
Uses: Progestational agent	X

AAP: Maternal medication usually compatible with breastfeeding

T½= ; **RID=** ; **Oral =** ; **MW=** 298

Clinical: Norethynodrel is a synthetic progestational agent used in oral contraceptives. Limited or no effects on infant. May decrease volume of breastmilk to some degree in some mothers if therapy initiated too soon after birth and if dose is too high. See norethindrone, medroxyprogesterone.

NORFLOXACIN; *Noroxin*	L3
Uses: Fluoroquinolone antibiotic	C

AAP: Not reviewed

T½= 3.3 hours; **RID=** ; **Oral =** 30-40%; **MW=** 319

Clinical: Although other members in the fluoroquinolone family are secreted into breastmilk (see ciprofloxacin, ofloxacin), only limited data are available on this drug. Wise has suggested that norfloxacin is not present in breastmilk. The manufacturer's product information states that doses of 200 mg do not produce detectable concentrations in milk although this was a single dose. Of the fluoroquinolone family, norfloxacin, levofloxacin, or perhaps ofloxacin may be preferred over others for use in a breastfeeding mother.

NORTRIPTYLINE; *Aventyl, Pamelor, Norventyl, Apo-Nortriptyline*	L2
Uses: Tricyclic antidepressant	D

AAP: Drugs whose effect on nursing infants is unknown but may be of concern

T½= 16-90 hours; **RID=** 1.7% - 3.1%; **Oral =** 51%; **MW=** 263

Clinical: Nortriptyline is a tricyclic antidepressant and is the active metabolite of amitriptyline (Elavil). A pooled analysis of 35 studies with an average dose of 78 mg/day reported a detectable level of nortriptyline in breast milk in only one patient, with a concentration of 230 ng/mL. The authors suggest that breastfeeding infants exposed to nortriptyline are unlikely to develop detectable concentrations in plasma, and therefore breastfeeding during nortriptyline therapy is not contraindicated.

NYSTATIN; *Mycostatin, Nilstat, Nadostine, Candistatin*	L1
Uses: Antifungal	B

AAP: Not reviewed

T½= ; **RID=** ; **Oral** = Poor; **MW=**

Clinical: Nystatin is safe to use during breastfeeding. It is poorly absorbed orally, and plasma levels are undetectable. Transfer to breast milk is highly unlikely.

OCTREOTIDE ACETATE AND [111]-INDIUM OCTREOTIDE; *Sandostatin LAR, OctreoScan, [111]-Indium Octreotide, Octreotide Acetate*	L3
Uses: Somatostatin analog	B

AAP: Not reviewed

T½= 1.7 hours; **RID=** ; **Oral** = 0.15; **MW=** 1019

Clinical: The oral bioavailability of octreotide is probably nil and would not pose a problem for a breastfeeding infant. Radioactivity leaves the plasma rapidly; one third of the radioactive injected dose remains in the blood pool at 10 minutes after administration. Plasma levels continue to decline so that by 20 hours post-injection, about 1% of the radioactive dose is found in the blood pool. The biological half-life of indium In-[111] pentetreotide is 6 hours. Half of the injected dose is recoverable in urine within six hours after injection, 85% is recovered in the first 24 hours, and over 90% is recovered in urine by two days. Hepatobiliary excretion represents a minor route of elimination, and less than 2% of the injected dose is recovered in feces within three days after injection. The return to breastfeeding is largely dependent on the dose, but 3 days would largely eliminate any risks at the lower dose.

OFLOXACIN; *Floxin, Ocuflox*	L2
Uses: Fluoroquinolone antibiotic	C

AAP: Maternal medication usually compatible with breastfeeding

T½= 5-7 hours; **RID=** 3.1%; **Oral** = 98 %; **MW=** 361

Clinical: Ofloxacin is a typical fluoroquinolone antimicrobial. Breastmilk concentrations are reported equal to maternal plasma levels. In one study in lactating women who received 400 mg oral doses twice daily, drug concentrations in breastmilk averaged 0.05-2.41 mg/L in milk (24 hours and 2 hours post-dose respectively). The only probably risk is a change in gut flora, diarrhea, and a remote risk of overgrowth of C. Difficile. Ofloxacin levels in breastmilk are consistently lower (37%) than ciprofloxacin. If a fluoroquinolone is required, ofloxacin, levofloxacin, or norfloxacin are probably the better choices for breastfeeding mothers.

OLANZAPINE; *Zyprexa, Symbyax, Zyprexa Relprevv*	L2
Uses: Antipsychotic	C

AAP: Not reviewed

T½= 21-54 hours; **RID=** 1.2%; **Oral** = >57%; **MW=** 312

Clinical: Olanzapine is an atypical antipsychotic agent structurally similar to clozapine and may be used for treating schizophrenia. In a recent and excellent study of seven mother-infant nursing pairs levels in milk were low and olanzapine was undetected in the plasma of six infants tested. All infants were healthy and experienced no observable side effects. The maximum relative infant dose was approximately 1.2%.

OLMESARTAN MEDOXOMIL; *Benicar, Benicar HCT*	L3
Uses: Antihypertensive	C

AAP: Not reviewed

T½= 13 hours; **RID=** ; **Oral** = 26%; **MW=** 558

Clinical: Olmesartan (Benicar) and Olmesartan plus Hydrochlorothiazide (Benicar HCT) are antihypertensives. Olmesartan is an angiotensin II receptor antagonist and hydrochlorothiazide is a diuretic. Olmesartan medoxomil is a prodrug and is rapidly metabolized in the GI tract to the active Olmesartan antihypertensive. It affectively blocks the angiotensin II receptor site. While it is different from the ACE inhibitors, it effectively produces the same end result, hypotension. Use in pregnancy is contraindicated. No data are available on its transfer to human milk, but its use in newborn infants could be risky.

OLOPATADINE OPHTHALMIC; *Patanol*	L2
Uses: Ophthalmic antihistamine	C

AAP: Not reviewed

T½= 3 hours; **RID=** ; **Oral =** ; **MW=** 373

Clinical: Olopatadine is a selective H1-receptor antagonist and inhibitor of histamine release from mast cells. It is used topically in the eye. Kinetic studies by the manufacturer suggest that absorption is low in adults and that plasma levels are undetectable in most cases (<0.5 ng/mL). Samples in which olopatadine was found in the plasma compartment were at 2 hours and were <1.3 ng/mL. Because adult plasma levels are so low, it is extremely unlikely any would be detectable in human milk. No data are available reporting levels in human milk but the risk is probably quite low.

OLSALAZINE; *Dipentum*	L3
Uses: Antiinflammatory	C

AAP: Not reviewed

T½= 0.9 hours; **RID=** 0.9%; **Oral =** 2.4% (olsalazine); **MW=** 346

Clinical: Transfer of olsalazine into human milk is minimal since it is highly protein bound, has a short half-life, and has a very low oral absorption rate. Breastfeeding while taking olsalazine poses little risk to the infant. Some diarrhea and cramping may occur in the breastfed infant after prolonged exposure.

OMALIZUMAB; *Xolair*	L3
Uses: Monoclonal antibody	B

AAP: Not reviewed

T½= 26 days; **RID=** ; **Oral =** 62%; **MW=** 149,000

Clinical: Omalizumab (Xolair) is used to treat persistent allergic asthma that cannot be controlled using inhaled corticosteroids. It works by inhibiting IgE binding to the receptor on mast cells and basophils, in turn decreasing the release of mediators in the allergic response. The manufacturer suggests that omalizumab may be secreted into human breastmilk based on monkey studies where milk levels were only 1.5% of maternal blood levels, which would be exceedingly low. However, no studies have been performed in humans. This product would not be orally bioavailable in an infant.

OMEPRAZOLE; *Prilosec, Zegerid OTC, Losec*	L2
Uses: Reduces gastric acid secretion	C

AAP: Not reviewed

T½= 1 hr.; **RID=** 1.1%; **Oral** = 30-40%; **MW=** 345

Clinical: Omeprazole poses little risk to a breastfeeding infant. Levels in milk are low, and it is unstable in the stomach at low pH. Virtually all omeprazole ingested via milk would probably be destroyed in the stomach of the infant prior to absorption.

ONDANSETRON; *Zofran, Zuplenz*	L2
Uses: Antiemetic	B

AAP: Not reviewed

T½= 3.6 hours; **RID=** ; **Oral** = 56-66%; **MW=** 293

Clinical: Ondansetron is used clinically for reducing the nausea and vomiting associated with chemotherapy. It has occasionally been used during pregnancy without effect on the fetus. It is available for oral and IV administration. Ondansetron is secreted in animal milk, but no data on humans is available. Four studies of ondansetron use in pediatric patients 4-18 years of age are available.

ORLISTAT; *Xenical, Alli*	L3
Uses: Lipase inhibitor	B

AAP: Not reviewed

T½= 1-2 hours; **RID=** ; **Oral** = minimal; **MW=** 495

Clinical: Orlistat, now available over the counter as well as prescription, is used in the management of obesity. It is a reversible inhibitor of gastric and pancreatic lipases, thus it inhibits absorption of dietary fats by 30%. No studies have been performed on the transmission of orlistat into the breastmilk. With high protein binding, moderately high molecular weight, and poor oral absorption, it is unlikely that orlistat would enter breastmilk in clinically relevant amounts, or affect a breastfeeding infant. However, due to orlistat's effect on the absorption of fat soluble vitamins and other fats, nutritional status of a breastfeeding mother should be closely monitored.

ORPHENADRINE CITRATE; *Norflex, Banflex, Norgesic, Flexon, Disipal, Orfenace*	L3
Uses: Muscle relaxant	C
AAP: Not reviewed	
T½= 14 hours; **RID=** ; **Oral** = 95%; **MW=** 269	
Clinical: Orphenadrine is an analog of Benadryl. It is primarily used as a muscle relaxant although its primary effects are anticholinergic. No data is available on its secretion into breastmilk.	

OSELTAMIVIR PHOSPHATE; *Tamiflu*	L2
Uses: Anti-viral for influenza A and B	C
AAP: Not reviewed	
T½= 6-10 hours; **RID=** 0.5%; **Oral** = 75%; **MW=** 312	
Clinical: The transfer of Oseltamivir into human milk is incredibly low because plasma levels are low. Data from one patient suggests relative infant dose of 0.5%. This product is probably of minimal risk to a breastfed infant. It has recently been recommended for use in breastfeeding mothers by the CDC.	

OSMOTIC LAXATIVES; *Milk of Magnesia, Fleet Phospho-Soda, Citrate of Magnesia, Epsom Salt, Acilac, Citromag*	L1
Uses: Laxatives	C
AAP: Not reviewed	
T½= ; **RID=** ; **Oral** = Poor; **MW=**	
Clinical: Osmotic or Saline laxatives comprise a large number of magnesium and phosphate compounds, but all work similarly in that they osmotically pull and retain water in the GI tract, thus functioning as laxatives. Because they are poorly absorbed, they largely stay in the GI tract and are eliminated without significant systemic absorption. The small amount of magnesium and phosphate salts absorbed are rapidly cleared by the kidneys. Products considered osmotic laxatives include: Milk of Magnesia, Epsom Salts, Citrate of Magnesia, Fleets Phospho-soda, and other sodium phosphate compounds.	

OXAPROZIN; *Daypro*	L3
Uses: Nonsteroidal analgesic	C

AAP: Not reviewed

T½= 42-50 hours; **RID=** ; **Oral =** 95%; **MW=** 293

Clinical: Oxaprozin belongs to the NSAID family of analgesics and is reputed to have lesser GI side effects than certain others. Although its long half-life could prove troublesome in breastfed infants, it is probably poorly transferred to human milk. No data on transfer into human milk are available although it is known to transfer into animal milk.

OXAZEPAM; *Serax, Apo-Oxazepam, Novoxapam, Zapex*	L3
Uses: Benzodiazepine antianxiety drug	D

AAP: Not reviewed

T½= 12 hours; **RID=** 1%; **Oral =** 97%; **MW=** 287

Clinical: Oxazepam is a typical benzodiazepine (See Valium) and is used in anxiety disorders. Of the benzodiazepines, oxazepam is the least lipid soluble, which accounts for its low levels in milk. In one study of a patient receiving 10 mg three times daily for 3 days, the concentration of oxazepam in breastmilk was relatively constant between 24 and 30 µg/L from the evening of the first day. The milk/plasma ratio ranged from 0.1 to 0.33.

OXCARBAZEPINE; *Trileptal*	L3
Uses: Anticonvulsant	C

AAP: Not reviewed

T½= 9 hours MHD; **RID=** ; **Oral =** Complete; **MW=** 252

Clinical: Oxcarbazepine is used in the treatment of partial seizures in adults and as adjunctive therapy in the treatment of partial seizures in children. In a brief and somewhat incomplete study of a pregnant patient who received 300 mg three times daily while pregnant, plasma levels were studied in her infant for the first 5 days postpartum while the infant was breastfeeding. While no breastmilk levels were reported, plasma levels of this drug were essentially the same as the mothers immediately after delivery, suggesting complete transfer transplacentally of the drug. However, while breastfeeding for the next 5 days, plasma levels of MHD in the infant declined significantly. No neonatal side effects were reported by the authors.

OXYBUTYNIN; *Ditropan, Apo-Oxybutynin, Oxybutyn*	L3
Uses: Anticholinergic, antispasmodic	B

AAP: Not reviewed

T½= 1-2 hours; **RID=** ; **Oral** = 6%; **MW=** 393

Clinical: Oxybutynin is an anticholinergic agent used to provide antispasmodic effects for conditions characterized by involuntary bladder spasms and reduces urinary urgency and frequency. Oxybutynin is a tertiary amine which is poorly absorbed orally (only 6%). Further, the maximum plasma levels (Cmax) generally attained are less than 31.7 nanogram/mL. Levels in milk are unpublished but likely low.

OXYCODONE; *Tylox, Percodan, OxyContin, Roxicet, Endocet, Roxiprin, Percocet, Supeudol*	L3
Uses: Narcotic analgesic	B

AAP: Not reviewed

T½= 3-6 hours; **RID=** 3.5%; **Oral** = 50%; **MW=** 315

Clinical: Oxycodone is secreted and may concentrate in milk. There have been no untoward effects in breastfed infants. Observe for sedation and withdrawal symptoms.

OXYMETAZOLINE; *Afrin Original Spray, Dristan 12 Hour Nasal Spray, Zicam Intense Sinus Relief*	L3
Uses: OTC active ingredient	

AAP: Not reviewed

T½= 5-8 hours; **RID=** ; **Oral** = ; **MW=** 260.7

Clinical: Oxymetazoline is the preferred decongestant for use in breastfeeding as it has minimal absorption and is given intranasally. Does not decrease milk production like pseudoephedrine.

OXYMORPHONE; *Numorphane, Opana*	L3
Uses: Opiate analgesic	C

AAP: Not reviewed

T½= 7.8 hours (oral); **RID=** ; **Oral** = 10%; **MW=** 337

Clinical: Oxymorphone is a potent opioid analgesic used to treat moderate to severe pain. On a weight basis, it is 8-10 times more potent than morphine, and it may produce more nausea and vomiting, but less constipation than morphine. It differs from morphine in its effects in that it generates less euphoria, sedation, itching and other histamine effects and it has no antitussive properties. It is poorly absorbed orally. Milk levels are as yet unreported. However, some caution is recommended with the prolonged use of this opioid analgesic.

OXYTOCIN; *Pitocin, Toesen*	L2
Uses: Labor induction	X
AAP: Not reviewed	
T½= 3-5 minutes; **RID**= ; **Oral** = Minimal; **MW**= >1000	

Clinical: Oxytocin is obviously required for letdown in breastfeeding mothers and it could potentially be useful in those mothers who are apparently unable to let down their milk. Available as an intranasal spray, it has been used for years in Europe and other countries where the intranasal product is available.

PANTOPRAZOLE; *Protonix, Pantoloc*	L1
Uses: Suppresses gastric acid production	B
AAP: Not reviewed	
T½= 1.5 hour; **RID**= 0.9%; **Oral** = 77% Enteric coated; **MW**= 383	

Clinical: Levels in milk were very low and were undetectable after 4 hours. Pantoprazole is unstable at pH less than 4.0. Virtually none would be absorbed.

PANTOTHENIC ACID	L1
Uses: Vitamin B-5	A
AAP: Not reviewed	
T½= ; **RID**= ; **Oral** = ; **MW**= 219	

Clinical: Pantothenic acid, or vitamin B-5, is needed to form coenzyme-A, which is a carrier carbon within the cell. Pantothenic acid is often used in high doses in excess of 10 g/day for the treatment of acne. The recommended daily allowance for pregnant women is 6 mg/day, while breastfeeding women need 7 mg/day. The recommended dose for infants less than 6 months is 1.7 mg/day, while infants over 6 months are to receive 2 mg/day. No adverse effects from oral administration of higher oral dosages of pantothenic acid were found. Concentrations found in milk are between 2 and 2.5 mg/L, with a weak correlation between maternal intake and milk levels. This would correspond to a daily dose of around 0.33-0.375 mg/kg/day for breastfeeding infants.

PAROXETINE; *Paxil*	L2
Uses: Antidepressant, serotonin reuptake inhibitor	D

AAP: Drugs whose effect on nursing infants is unknown but may be of concern

T½= 21 hours; **RID=** 1.2% - 2.8%; **Oral** = Complete; **MW=** 329

Clinical: Levels in milk are quite low and average less than 2.8% of the maternal dose. Probably quite safe in breastfeeding mothers. If used during pregnancy, expect neonatal withdrawal syndrome postpartum.

PARVOVIRUS B19	L3
Uses:	

AAP: Not reviewed

T½= ; **RID=** ; **Oral** = ; **MW=**

Clinical: The virus is seen in breastmilk, but transmission is very rare. It seems that the highest risk is during an infection at the time of birth. At this time, the breastmilk has a high titer of virus and no antibodies to neutralize the virus.

PEGAPTANIB SODIUM; *Macugen*	L3
Uses: Angiogenesis inhibitor	B

AAP: Not reviewed

T½= 10 days; **RID=** ; **Oral** = Nil; **MW=** 50,000

Clinical: This large polymer is slowly absorbed follywing intravitreous administration. Plasma levels are exceedingly low (80 ng/mL following a 3 mg dose. It would be exceedingly unlikely this large polymer would ever enter the milk compartment, or be orally bioavailable. There have been no studies performed to measure the levels in human milk. It would be exceedingly unlikely this large polymer would ever enter the milk compartment, or be orally bioavailable.

PEGFILGRASTIM; *Neulasta*	L3
Uses: Colony stimulating factor	C
AAP: Not reviewed	

T½= 15-80 hours; **RID=** ; **Oral** = Nil; **MW=** 39,000

Clinical: Probably too large to enter milk after the colostral period. It would not likely be orally bioavailable. There are no reported levels in human milk. Due to large molecular weight of this drug, milk levels and oral bioavailability are likely to be low. Lactation studies in rodents did not show any untoward effects on growth and development of breastfed rodents.

PENCICLOVIR; *Denavir*	L3
Uses: Antiviral agent	B
AAP: Not reviewed	

T½= 2.3 hours; **RID=** ; **Oral** = 1.5%; **MW=**

Clinical: Penciclovir is an antiviral agent for the treatment of cold sores (herpes simplex labialis) of the lips and face and occasionally for herpes zoster (Shingles). Following topical administration, plasma levels are undetectable. Because oral bioavailability is nil and maternal plasma levels are undetectable following topical therapy, it is extremely unlikely that detectable amounts would transfer into human milk or be absorbable by an infant.

PENICILLAMINE; *Cuprimine, Depen*	L4
Uses: Used in arthritis, autoimmune syndromes	D
AAP: Not reviewed	

T½= 1.7-3.2 hours; **RID=** ; **Oral** = Complete; **MW=** 149

Clinical: Penicillamine is a potent chelating agent used to chelate copper, iron, mercury, lead, and other metals. It is also used to suppress the immune response in rheumatoid arthritis and other immunologic syndromes. It is extremely dangerous during pregnancy. Safety has not been established during lactation. Penicillamine is a potent drug that requires constant observation and care by attending physicians. Recommend discontinuing lactation if this drug is mandatory.

PENICILLIN G; *Pfizerpen, Crystapen, Megacillin, Bicillin L-A, Ayercillin*	L1
Uses: Antibiotic	B

AAP: Maternal medication usually compatible with breastfeeding

T½= <1.5 hours; **RID**= ; **Oral** = 15-30%; **MW**= 372

Clinical: Penicillin is safe to use during breastfeeding. Milk levels are low and pose little risk to the infant. Observe for diarrhea, rash, and hypersensitivity to penicillin in the breastfed infant. Compatible with breastfeeding in non-hypersensitive infants.

PENTAZOCINE; *Talwin, Talacen*	L3
Uses: Analgesic	C

AAP: Not reviewed

T½= 2-3 hours; **RID**= ; **Oral** = 18%; **MW**= 285

Clinical: Pentazocine is a synthetic opiate and is also an opiate antagonist. Once absorbed it undergoes extensive hepatic metabolism and only small amounts achieve plasma levels. It is primarily used as a mild analgesic. No data is available on transfer into breastmilk.

PENTOBARBITAL; *Nembutol, Nova-Rectal, Novo-Pentobarb*	L3
Uses: Sedative, hypnotic	D

AAP: Not reviewed

T½= 15-50 hours; **RID**= 1.8%; **Oral** = 95%; **MW**= 248

Clinical: Pentobarbital is a short acting barbiturate primarily used at a sedative. Following a dose of 100 mg for 3 days, the concentration of pentobarbital 19 hours after the last dose was 0.17 mg/L. The effect of short acting barbiturates on the breastfed infant is unknown, but significant tolerance and addiction can occur. Use caution if used in large amounts. No reported harmful effects breastfeeding infants.

PENTOSAN POLYSULFATE; *Elmiron.*	L2
Uses: Urinary tract analgesic	B
AAP: Not reviewed	

T½= <5 hours; **RID=** ; **Oral** = 3%; **MW=** 6000

Clinical: Pentosan polysulfate is a negatively-charged synthetic sulfated polysaccharide with Heparin-like properties although it is used as a urinary tract analgesic for interstitial cystitis. It is structurally related to dextran sulfate with a molecular weight of 4000-6000 daltons. Oral bioavailability is low, only 6% is absorbed systemically. Pentosan adheres to the bladder wall mucosa and may act as a buffer to control cell permeability preventing irritating solutes in the urine from reaching the cell membrane. Although no data are available on its transfer into human milk, its large molecular weight and its poor oral bioavailability would largely preclude the transfer and absorption of clinically relevant amounts in breastfed infants.

PENTOXIFYLLINE; *Trental, Apo-Pentoxifylline*	L2
Uses: Reduces blood viscosity	C
AAP: Not reviewed	

T½= 0.4-1.6 hours; **RID=** 0.2%; **Oral** = Complete; **MW=** 278

Clinical: Pentoxifylline and its metabolites improve the flow properties of blood by decreasing its viscosity. It is a methylxanthine derivative similar in structure to caffeine and is extensively metabolized although the metabolites do not have long half-lives. In a group of 5 breastfeeding women who received a single 400 mg dose, the mean milk/plasma ratio was 0.87 for the parent compound. The milk/plasma ratios for the metabolites were lower: 0.54, 0.76, and 1.13. Average milk concentration at 2 hours following the dose was 73.9 μg/L.

PERFLUTREN PROTEIN TYPE A; *Optison, Definity*   L3

Uses: Diagnostic agent   C

AAP: Not reviewed

T½= 1.3 minutes; **RID=** ; **Oral =** Nil; **MW=**

Clinical: Perflutren protein type A is a unique contrast agent used in patients with suboptimal echocardiograms to make the left ventricular chamber opaque. This product releases perflutren gas molecules that are completely eliminated in the human lung in 10 minutes. Perflutren gas is not metabolized but passes rapidly from the body. Although there are no data on levels in human milk, this product is so rapidly dissipated, that the risk to the infant would be nil.

PERMETHRIN; *Nix, Elimite, A-200, Pyrinex, Pyrinyl, Acticin*   L2

Uses: Insecticide, scabicide   B

AAP: Not reviewed

T½= ; **RID=** ; **Oral =** ; **MW=** 391

To use, recommend that the hair be washed with detergent, and then saturated with permethrin liquid for 10 minutes before rinsing with water. One treatment is all that is required. At 14 days, a second treatment may be required if viable lice are seen. Elimite cream is generally recommended for scabies infestations and should be applied head to toe for 8-12 hours in infants, and body (not head) only in adults. Reapplication may be needed in 7 days if live mites appear.

PERPHENAZINE AND AMITRIPTYLINE; *Triavil, Etrafon*   L3

Uses: Phenothiazine antipsychotic and antidepressant   C

AAP: Drugs whose effect on nursing infants is unknown but may be of concern

T½= 8-12 hours; **RID=** 0.1%; **Oral =** Complete; **MW=** 403

Clinical: Commonly combined in the USA with amitriptyline it is called Etrafon or Triavil. For information on amitriptyline see individual monograph. Perphenazine is a phenothiazine derivative used as an antipsychotic or sedative. In a study of one patient receiving either 16 or 24 mg/day of perphenazine divided in two doses at 12 hour intervals, milk levels were 2.1 µg/L and 3.2 µg/L respectively. The authors estimate the dose to be approximately 0.1% of the weight-adjusted maternal dose. The authors report that during a 3 month exposure, the infant thrived and had no adverse response to the medication.

PHENAZOPYRIDINE HCL; *Pyridium, Eridium, Azo-Standard, Azo-Diac, Phenazo, Pyronium*	L3
Uses: Urinary tract analgesic	B
AAP: Not reviewed	

T½= ; RID= ; Oral = Complete; **MW=** 250

Clinical: Phenazopyridine is an azo dye that is rapidly excreted in the urine, where it exerts a topical analgesic effect on urinary tract mucosa. Pyridium is only moderately effective and produces a reddish-orange discoloration of the urine. It may also ruin contact lenses. It is not known if Pyridium transfers into breastmilk, but it probably does to a limited degree. This product, due to limited efficacy, should probably not be used in lactating women although it is doubtful that it would be harmful to an infant. This product is highly colored and can stain clothing. Stains can be removed by soaking in a solution of 0.25% sodium dithionite.

PHENCYCLIDINE; *PCP, Angel Dust*	L5
Uses: Hallucinogen	X
AAP: Drugs of abuse for which adverse effects have been reported	

T½= 24-51 hours; **RID= ; Oral =** Complete; **MW=** 243

Clinical: Phencyclidine, also called Angel Dust, is a potent and extremely dangerous hallucinogen. High concentrations are secreted into breastmilk (>10 times plasma level) of mice. Continued secretion into milk occurs over long periods of time (perhaps months). One patient who consumed PCP 41 days prior to lactating had a milk level of 3.90 µg/L.

EXTREMELY DANGEROUS TO NURSING INFANT. PCP is stored for long periods in adipose tissue. Urine samples are positive for 14-30 days in adults and probably longer in infants. The infant could test positive for PCP long after maternal exposure, particularly if breastfeeding. Definitely contraindicated.

PHENIRAMINE; *Avil, Daneral, Inhiston, Trimeton, Tripoton*	L3
Uses: Antihistamine	A
AAP: Not reviewed	
T½= ; **RID=** ; **Oral =** ; **MW=** 240.3434	
Clinical: There are no adequate and well-controlled studies or case reports in breastfeeding women. May induce sedation, recommend non-sedating antihistamines (Zyrtec, Claritin, Allegra).	

PHENOBARBITAL; *Luminal, Barbilixir*	L3
Uses: Long acting barbiturate sedative, anticonvulsant	D
AAP: Drugs associated with significant side effects and should be given with caution	
T½= 53-140 hours; **RID=** 24%; **Oral =** 80% (Adult); **MW=** 232	
Clinical: Phenobarbital is a long half-life barbiturate frequently used as an anticonvulsant in adults and during the neonatal period. The half-life in premature infants can be extremely long (100-500 hours) and plasma levels must be closely monitored. Although varied, milk/plasma ratios vary from 0.46 to 0.6. Baby will receive 1/3 of mother's dose; observe for apnea, sedation. Possibility of withdrawal symptoms such as jitteriness, irritability, crying, sweating when drug withdrawn. Baby's blood levels should be monitored if mother on long term therapy.	

PHENTERMINE; *Fastin, Zantryl, Ionamin, Adipex-P*	**L4**
Uses: Appetite suppressant	**C**
AAP: Not reviewed	
T½= 7-20 hours; **RID=** ; **Oral =** Complete; **MW=** 149	

Clinical: Phentermine is an appetite suppressant structurally similar to the amphetamine family. As such it frequently produces CNS stimulation. No data is available on transfer to human milk. This product has a very small molecular weight (149) and would probably transfer into human milk in significant quantities and could product stimulation, anorexia, tremors, and other CNS side effects in the newborn. The use of this product in breastfeeding mothers would be difficult to justify and is not advised.

PHENYLEPHRINE; *Neo-Synephrine, AK-Dilate, Vicks Sinex Nasal, Neofrin, Mydfrin, Dionephrine*	**L3**
Uses: Decongestant	**C**
AAP: Not reviewed	
T½= 2-3 hours; **RID=** ; **Oral =** 38%; **MW=** 203	

Clinical: Phenylephrine is probably okay to use during breastfeeding since it is poorly oral absorbed. Although there are some concerns for decreased milk production similar to pseudoephedrine, especially in late-lactating mothers (breastfeeding longer than a year). A suitable decongestant in breastfeeding is oxymetazoline.

PHENYLPROPANOLAMINE; *Dexatrim, Acutrim, Caldomine-DH*	**L2**
Uses: Adrenergic, nasal decongestant, anorexiant	**C**
AAP: Not reviewed	
T½= 5.6 hours; **RID=** ; **Oral =** 100%; **MW=** 188	

Clinical: Phenylpropanolamine is an adrenergic compound frequently used in nasal decongestants and also diet pills. It produces significant constriction of nasal mucosa and is a common ingredient in cold preparations. No data are available on its secretion into human milk, but due to its low molecular weight and its rapid entry past the blood-brain-barrier, it should be expected. It has recently been withdrawn from the US market.

PHENYLTOLOXAMINE; *Percogesic, Dologesic, Flextra-650*	L3
Uses: Antihistamine/analgesic	C
AAP: Not reviewed	
T½= ; **RID**= ; **Oral** = well absorbed; **MW**= 255	
Clinical: Phenyltoloxamine is an antihistamine with analgesic and antitussive properties used in over-the-counter preparations. No data are available on the transfer of this antihistamine into human milk. Similar to Benadryl, this old product should not normally be used in breastfeeding mothers, although it is probably compatible with breastfeeding.	

PHENYTOIN; *Dilantin, Novo-Phenytoin*	L2
Uses: Anticonvulsant	D
AAP: Maternal medication usually compatible with breastfeeding	
T½= 6-24 hours; **RID**= 0.6% - 7.7%; **Oral** = 70-100%; **MW**= 252	
Clinical: The transfer of phenytoin into human milk seems to be low in most of the studies available, and no untoward effects to the infants were reported. Although occurrence is rare, observe for drowsiness or poor suckling, To minimize harm to the infant, a lower maternal dose is advised. The neonatal half-life of phenytoin is highly variable for the first week of life. Monitoring of the infants' plasma may be useful although it is not definitely required. All of the current studies indicate rather low levels of phenytoin in breastmilk and minimal plasma levels in breastfeeding infants.	

PHYTONADIONE; *Phytonadione, AquaMEPHYTON, Konakion, Mephyton, Vitamin K1*	L1
Uses: Vitamin K1	C
AAP: Maternal medication usually compatible with breastfeeding	
T½= ; **RID**= ; **Oral** = Complete; **MW**= 450	

Clinical: Vitamin K1 is often used to reverse the effects of oral anticoagulants and to prevent hemorrhagic disease of the newborn (HDN). It is used postnatally to preven neonatal hemorage in the brain. A single IM injection of 0.5 to 1 mg or an oral dose of 1-2 mg during the neonatal period is recommended by the AAP. Although controversial, it is generally recognized that exclusive breastfeeding may not provide sufficient vitamin K1 to provide normal clotting factors, particularly in the premature infant or those with malabsorptive disorders. Although vitamin K is transferred to human milk, the amount may not be sufficient to prevent hemorrhagic disease of the newborn. Vitamin K requires the presence of bile and other factors for absorption, and neonatal absorption may be slow or delayed due to the lack of requisite gut factors.

PILOCARPINE; *Isopto Carpine, Pilocar, Akarpine, Ocusert Pilo, Minims Pilocarpine*	L3
Uses: Intraocular hypotensive	C
AAP: Not reviewed	

T½= 0.76-1.55 hours; **RID=** ; **Oral** = Good; **MW=** 208

Clinical: Pilocarpine is a direct acting cholinergic agent used primarily in the eyes for treatment of open-angle glaucoma. The ophthalmic dose is approximately 1 mg or less per day, while the oral adult dose is approximately 15-30 mg daily. It is not known if pilocarpine enters milk, but it probably does in low levels due to its minimal plasma level. It is not likely that an infant would receive a clinical dose via milk, but this is presently unknown. Side effects would largely include diarrhea, gastric upset, excessive salivation, and other typical cholinergic symptoms.

PIMECROLIMUS; *Elidel*	L2
Uses: Cytokine inhibitor used for atopic dermatitis	C
AAP: Not reviewed	

T½= ; **RID=** ; **Oral** = Moderate; **MW=** 810

Clinical: Pimecrolimus is a topical agent used as a cytokine inhibitor for atopic dermatitis. Systemic absorption following topical application is minimal with reported blood concentrations consistently below 0.5 ng/milliliter following twice-daily application of the 1% cream. Oral absorption is unreported but probably low to moderate as plasma levels of 54 ng/mL have been reported following twice daily oral doses of 30 mg. Pimecrolimus is cleared for use in pediatric patients 2 years and older. No data are available on its transfer to human milk, but because the maternal plasma levels are so low, it is extremely remote that this agent would penetrate milk in clinically relevant amounts. However, its use on or around the nipples should be avoided as the clinical dose absorbed orally in the infant could be significant.

PIMOZIDE; *Orap*	L4
Uses: Potent tranquilizer	C
AAP: Not reviewed	
T½= 55 hours; **RID**= ; **Oral** = >50%; **MW**= 462	

Clinical: Pimozide is a potent neuroleptic agent primarily used for Tourette's syndrome and chronic schizophrenia which induces a low degree of sedation. No data are available on the secretion of pimozide into breastmilk. This is a highly risky product and numerous other antipsychotics are available. So this product is probably not worth the risk to the infant.

PIOGLITAZONE; *Actos*	L3
Uses: Oral antidiabetic agent	C
AAP: Not reviewed	
T½= 16-24 hours; **RID**= ; **Oral** = ; **MW**= 392	

Clinical: Pioglitazone is a thiazolidinediones family oral antidiabetic agent similar to troglitazone and rosiglitazone. It acts primarily by increasing insulin receptor sensitivity. In essence, the insulin receptor is activated reducing insulin resistance. This family also decreases hepatic gluconeogenesis and increases insulin-dependent muscle glucose uptake. They do not increase the release or secretion of insulin. No data are available on its entry into human milk.

PIPERACILLIN-TAZOBACTAM; *Zosyn*	L3
Uses: Anti bacterial	B

AAP: Not reviewed

T½= ; **RID=** ; **Oral =** ; **MW=**

Clinical: Piperacillin is an extended-spectrum penicillin. It is not absorbed orally and must be given IM or IV. Piperacillin when combined with tazobactam sodium is called Zosyn. Tazobactam is a penicillin-like inhibitor of the enzyme beta lactamase and has few clinical effects. Concentrations of piperacillin secreted into milk are believed to be extremely low. Its poor oral absorption would limit its absorption. I've had one report that it turned the milk blue.

PIPERACILLIN; *Zosyn, Pipracil*	L2
Uses: Penicillin antibiotic	B

AAP: Not reviewed

T½= 0.6-1.3 hours; **RID=** ; **Oral =** Poor; **MW=** 518

Clinical: Piperacillin probably enters milk in low levels as with most penicillins. It is not absorbed orally. Concentrations of piperacillin secreted into milk are believed to be extremely low. Its poor oral absorption would limit its absorption. I've had one report that it turned the milk blue. The infant had no symptoms.

PIRBUTEROL ACETATE; *Maxair*	L2
Uses: Bronchodilator for asthmatics	C

AAP: Not reviewed

T½= 2-3 hours; **RID=** ; **Oral =** Complete; **MW=** 240

Clinical: Pirbuterol is a classic beta-2 drug (similar to albuterol) for dilating pulmonary bronchi in asthmatic patients. It is administered by inhalation and, occasionally, orally. Plasma levels are all but undetectable with normal inhaled doses. No data exists on levels in milk, but they would probably be minimal if administered via inhalation. Oral preparations would provide much higher plasma levels and would be associated with a higher risk for breastfeeding infants.

PIROXICAM; *Feldene, Apo-Piroxicam, Novo-Pirocam*	L2
Uses: Non-steroidal analgesic for arthritis	C

AAP: Maternal medication usually compatible with breastfeeding

T½= 30-86 hours; **RID=** 3.4% - 5.8%; **Oral =** Complete; **MW=** 331

Clinical: Piroxicam is a typical nonsteroidal antiinflammatory commonly used in arthritics. Levels in milk are somewhat low, about 0.22 mg/L at 2.5 hours after dose. Even though piroxicam has a very long half-life, this report suggests its use to be safe in breastfeeding mothers.

PNEUMOCOCCAL VACCINE; *Prevnar, Pneumovax 23, Prevnar 13, Pneumo 23, Pneumovax 23*	L1
Uses: Vaccine	C

AAP: Not reviewed

T½= ; **RID=** ; **Oral =** Nil; **MW=**

Clinical: This is a nonviable pneumococcal vaccine. The 23 strain vaccine is not even active in infants which is the reason it is not marketed for this use. There are few if any contraindications for its use in breastfeeding mothers. Although technically not approved for use in breastfeeding mothers, Prevnar 7 is recommended by the AAP for use in infants 2 months of age and older. The CDC also suggests Pneumovax is of minimal risk to a breastfeeding infant. Therefore it is unlikely to produce an untoward effect in a breastfed infant.

PODOFILOX; *Condylox, Podophyllotoxin*	L3
Uses: Antimitotic agent use topically for treatment of genital warts	C

AAP: Not reviewed

T½= 1-4.5 hours; **RID=** ; **Oral =** ; **MW=** 414

Clinical: Podofilox is a strong antimitotic agent used to treat genital warts and Condyloma acuminatum. If used in small amounts, plasma levels are virtually undetectable. However, if used in larger amounts and areas, plasma levels are detectable. It is probably relatively unlikely that this agent will enter milk avidly, however, it is so toxic to cells, that if present in milk it could be problematic. It would be advisable to limit exposure of breastfeeding mothers to this agent, and to wait at least 4 hours to breastfeed following its application. I'd suggest avoiding this product if at all possible during breastfeeding.

POLIDOCANOL; *Asclera*	L3
Uses: Sclerosing Agent	C

AAP: Not reviewed

T½= 1.5 hours; **RID=** ; **Oral =** ; **MW=** 580

Clinical: The adverse effects of using polidocanol are mainly local. One time treatment poses minimal harm to the infant, since the half-life is short and the effects are local. However, since the manufacturer has obtained little pharmacokinetic data, the effects are uncertain. There are no adequate and well-controlled studies or case reports in breastfeeding women.

POLYETHYLENE GLYCOL-ELECTROLYTE SOLUTIONS; *GoLYTELY, Col-Lav, Colovage, Colyte, OCL, PegLyte*	L3
Uses: Bowel evacuant	C

AAP: Not reviewed

T½= ; **RID=** ; **Oral** = None; **MW=**

Clinical: PEG laxatives are most likely safe to use during breastfeeding, as oral absorption is negligible. Transfer to milk is highly unlikely due to limited absorption. No adverse effects have been reported in breastfed infants. Observe for diarrhea. Although no data are available on transfer into human milk, it is highly unlikely that enough maternal absorption would occur to produce milk levels.

POLYMYXIN B SULFATE; *Polysporin, Bacitracin, Ak-Spore, Akorn, Aerosporin, Neosporin, Cortisporin, Aerosporin*	L2
Uses: Antibacterial	B

AAP: Not reviewed

T½= 6 hours; **RID=** ; **Oral** = Minimal; **MW=** Large

Clinical: Polymyxin B sulfate is generally regarded as safe to use during breastfeeding. Topical absorption systemically is minimal. If present in milk, oral absorption is also minimal since it would largely be destroyed by the acidity of the GI tract. If applied to the nipple, advise patient to use sparingly. No data are available on its transfer to human milk. However, when used topically it is very unlikely enough would be absorbed transcutaneously to produce plasma or milk levels. Orally, it would be largely destroyed by the gastric acid in the infant as it is very unstable in acidic milieu. When applied topically to nipples in small amounts it is unlikely to produce problems in a breastfed infant.

POTASSIUM IODIDE; *SSKI*	L4
Uses: Antithyroid agent, Expectorant	D

AAP: Not reviewed

T½= 6 hours (blood); **RID**= ; **Oral** = Complete; **MW**= 166

Clinical: Use potassium iodide with caution while breastfeeding. Potassium iodide is not recommended for use in breastfeeding women. Thyroid suppression is possible in the breastfed infant. Thyroid storm may be treated with propranolol and propythiouracil. Use with extreme caution if at all. Combined with the fact that it is a poor expectorant and that it is concentrated in breastmilk, it is not recommended in breastfeeding mothers. However, following treatment of thyroid storm, mothers should pump and discard milk for at least 24-48 hours.

POVIDONE IODIDE; *Betadine, Iodex, Operand, Pharmadine, Proviodine*	L4
Uses: Special chelated iodine antiseptic	D
AAP: Maternal medication usually compatible with breastfeeding	

T½= ; **RID**= ; **Oral** = Complete; **MW**=

Clinical: Povidone iodide is a chelated form of iodine. It is primarily used as an antiseptic and antimicrobial. When placed on the adult skin, very little is absorbed. When used intravaginally, significant and increased plasma levels of iodine have been documented. In a study of 62 pregnant women who used povidone-iodine douches, significant increases in plasma iodine were noted, and a seven fold increase in fetal thyroid iodine content was reported. Topical application to infants has resulted in significant absorption through the skin. Once plasma levels are attained in the mother, iodide rapidly sequester in human milk at high milk/plasma ratios. See potassium iodide. High oral iodine intake in mothers is documented to produce thyroid suppression in breastfed infants. Use with extreme caution or not at all. Repeated use of povidone iodide is not recommended in nursing mothers or their infants.

PRAMIPEXOLE; *Mirapex*	L4
Uses: Dopamine agonist for Parkinson's disease	C
AAP: Not reviewed	

T½= 8 hours; **RID**= ; **Oral** = >90%; **MW**= 302

Clinical: Pramipexole is a nonergot dopamine agonist for use in treating the symptoms of Parkinson's disease and restless leg syndrome. While rodent studies showed rather high levels in milk, rats studies simply don't correlate with humans. No human studies are available concerning levels in milk. Regardless, pramipexole is known to reduce the secretion of prolactin, and it is possible that it could significantly reduce milk synthesis. This product should probably not be used in breastfeeding mothers.

PRAMLINTIDE ACETATE; *Symlin*	L3
Uses: Antihyperglycemic agent for diabetics	C

AAP: Not reviewed

T½= 48 minutes; **RID=** ; **Oral =** 40% SC; **MW=** 3949

Clinical: The is a rather large peptide(3949 daltons) which is unlikely to enter milk in clinically relevant amounts after the first week postpartum, nor would it likely be orally bioavailable to the infant. Further it does not induce hypoglycemia by itself, but only when co-administered with insulin. It is unlikely the presence of this product in milk would harm a breastfeeding infant. Be slightly more cautious the first week postpartum before onset of mature milk. I do not think it would be contraindicated in breastfeeding infants, but we have no data yet and some caution is certainly recommended.

PRAVASTATIN; *Pravachol*	L3
Uses: Lowers blood cholesterol	X

AAP: Not reviewed

T½= 77 hours; **RID=** ; **Oral =** 17%; **MW=** 446

Clinical: Pravastatin belongs to the HMG-CoA reductase family of cholesterol lowering drugs. Small amounts are believed to be secreted into human milk but the levels were unreported. The effect on an infant is unknown, but it could reduce cholesterol synthesis. Atherosclerosis is a chronic process and discontinuation of lipid-lowering drugs during pregnancy and lactation should have little to no impact on the outcome of long-term therapy of primary hypercholesterolemia. Cholesterol and other products of cholesterol biosynthesis are essential components for fetal and neonatal development and the use of cholesterol-lowering drugs would not be advisable under any circumstances.

PRAZEPAM; *Centrax*	L3
Uses: Antianxiety agent	D

AAP: Drugs whose effect on nursing infants is unknown but may be of concern

T½= 30-100 hours; **RID=** ; **Oral** = Complete; **MW=** 325

Clinical: Prazepam is a typical benzodiazepine that belongs to Valium family. It has a long half-life in adults. Peak plasma level occurs 6 hours post-dose. An active metabolite with a longer half-life is produced. No data is available on transfer into human milk. Most benzodiazepines have high milk/plasma ratios and transfer into milk readily. Observe infant closely for sedation. See diazepam.

PRAZIQUANTEL; *Biltricide*	L2
Uses: Anthelmintic	B

AAP: Not reviewed

T½= 0.8-3 hours; **RID=** 0.05%; **Oral** = 80%; **MW=** 312

Clinical: Praziquantel is a trematodicide used for treatment of schistosome infections and infestations of liver flukes. Using the data in one study, the relative infant dose would be approximately 0.05% of the maternal dose in both groups. These values are probably too low to harm an infant.

PRAZOSIN; *Minipress, Apo-Prazo, Novo-Prazin*	L4
Uses: Strong antihypertensive	C

AAP: Not reviewed

T½= 2-3 hours; **RID=** ; **Oral** = ; **MW=** 383

Clinical: Prazosin is an antihypertensive. Antihypertensives may reduce breastmilk production and prazosin may do likewise. Others in this family (doxazosin) are known to concentrate in milk. Exercise extreme caution when administering to nursing mothers.

PREDNICARBATE; *Dermatop*	L3
Uses: High potency steroid ointment	C

AAP: Not reviewed

T½= ; **RID=** ; **Oral** = ; **MW=** 488

Clinical: Prednicarbate is a high potency steroid ointment. Its absorption via skin surfaces is exceedingly low, even in infants. Its oral absorption is not reported but would probably be equivalent to prednisolone, or high. If recommended for topical application on the nipple, other less potent steroids should be suggested, including hydrocortisone or triamcinolone. If applied to the nipple, only extremely small amounts should be applied. See appendix C for other steroid ointment choices.

PREDNISONE-PREDNISOLONE; *Prednisone, Prednisolone*	L2
Uses: Steroid, corticosteroid	C
AAP: Maternal medication usually compatible with breastfeeding	

T½= 24+ hours; **RID=** 1.8% - 5.3%; **Oral** = Complete; **MW=** 346

Clinical: Small amounts of prenisone-prednisolone are transferred to the breast milk, although it is probably safe in breastfeeding. There is concern of growth impairment in breastfed infants with high-dose prolonged steroid therapy. Recommend using low-dose therapy, inhaled, or high-dose short-term therapy when needed to minimize exposure. In small doses, most steroids are certainly not contraindicated in nursing mothers. Whenever possible use low-dose alternatives such as aerosols or inhalers. Following administration, wait at least 4 hours if possible prior to feeding infant to reduce exposure. With high doses (>40 mg/day), particularly for long periods, steroids could potentially produce problems in infant growth and development, although we have absolutely no data in this area, or which doses would pose problems. Brief applications of high dose steroids are probably not contraindicated as the overall exposure is low. With prolonged high dose therapy, the infant should be closely monitored for growth and development.

PREGABALIN; *Lyrica*	L3
Uses: Analgesic	C
AAP: Not reviewed	

T½= 6 hours; **RID=** ; **Oral** = 90%; **MW=** 159

Clinical: While there are no data on its transfer into human milk, it should be expected. Observe for sedation, constipation, etc. However, due to the kinetics of the drug, its passage into the milk compartment is probable, and its oral bioavailability to the infant would be high. Therefore, nursing mothers should use caution taking pregabalin while nursing.

PRIMAQUINE PHOSPHATE	L3
Uses: Antimalarial	C

AAP: Not reviewed

T½= 4-7 hours; **RID**= ; **Oral** = 96%; **MW**= 259

Clinical: Primaquine is a typical antimalarial medication. No data are available on its transfer into human milk. Maternal plasma levels are rather low, only 53-107 nanogram/mL, suggesting that milk levels might be rather low as well.

PRIMIDONE; *Mysoline, Apo-Primidone, Sertan*	L3
Uses: Anticonvulsant	D

AAP: Drugs associated with significant side effects and should be given with caution

T½= 10-21 hours (primidone); **RID**= 8.4% - 8.6%; **Oral** = 90%; **MW**= 218

Clinical: Primidone is excreted into breast milk, and may cause sedation in the breastfed infant during the neonatal period. Primidone is metabolized to phenobarbital, which accumulates chronically. Caution and close monitoring is advised. Some sedation has been reported, particularly during the neonatal period.

PROBENECID; *Benemid, Benecid, Probanalan, Probenecid, Proben, Apurina, Uricosid*	L2
Uses: Used in treatment of gout	C

AAP: Not reviewed

T½= 6-12 hours; **RID**= 0.7%; **Oral** = Complete; **MW**= 285

Clinical: Levels in milk are very low. RID = 0.7%. However, even small plasma levels in the infant might affect elimination rate kinetics of many drugs. Even though milk and infant plasma levels may be low, be cautious when using probenecid with other medications whose renal elimination may be profoundly affected by probenecid.

PROCAINAMIDE; *Pronestyl, Procan, Procan SR, Apo-Procainamide* | L3

Uses: Antiarrhythmic	C

AAP: Maternal medication usually compatible with breastfeeding

T½= 3.0 hours; **RID=** 5.4%; **Oral** = 75-90%; **MW=** 271

Clinical: Procainamide is an antiarrhythmic agent. Procainamide and its active metabolite are secreted into breastmilk in moderate concentrations. In one patient receiving 500 mg four times daily, the breast milk levels of procainamide at 0, 3, 6, 9, and 12 hours were 5.3, 3.9, 10.2, 4.8, and 2.6 mg/L respectively. The milk/serum ratio varied from 1.0 at 12 hours to 7.3 at 6 hours post-dose (mean= 4.3). The milk levels averaged 5.4 mg/L for parent drug and 3.5 mg/L for metabolite. Although levels in milk are still too small to provide significant blood levels in an infant, use with caution.

PROCAINE HCL; *Novocain* | L3

Uses: Local anesthetic	C

AAP: Not reviewed

T½= 7.7 minutes; **RID=** ; **Oral** = Poor; **MW=** 236

Clinical: Procaine is a local anesthetic with low potential for systemic toxicity and short duration of action. No data are available on its transfer to human milk, but it is unlikely. Most other local anesthetics (see bupivacaine, lidocaine) penetrate milk only poorly and it is likely that procaine, due to its brief plasma half-life, would produce even lower milk levels. Due to its ester bond, it would be poorly bioavailable.

PROCHLORPERAZINE; *Compazine, Prorazin, Stemetil, Nu-Prochlor* | L3

Uses: Antiemetic, tranquilizer-sedative	C

AAP: Not reviewed

T½= 10-20 hours; **RID=** ; **Oral** = Complete; **MW=** 374

Clinical: Prochlorperazine is a phenothiazine primarily used as an antiemetic in adults and pediatric patients. There are no data yet concerning breastmilk levels but other phenothiazine derivatives enter milk in small amounts. Because infants are extremely hypersensitive to these compounds, I suggest caution in younger infants. This product may also increase prolactin levels. See promethazine as a safer alternative, although neonatal apnea is a consistent problem with this family of drugs. Use with extreme caution in infants subject to apnea.

PROGESTERONE; *Crinone, Prometrium, Progesterone Vaginal Ring, Crinone, Gesterol*	L3
Uses: Progestational agent	B

AAP: Maternal medication usually compatible with breastfeeding

T½= 13-18 hours; **RID**= ; **Oral** = Low; **MW**= 314

Clinical: In some mothers oral progestins may suppress milk productions. Always warn moms to watch for lower milk production. Oral "progesterone" itself is hardly even absorbed so it is probably not a problem for breastfeeding mothers. Intravaginal preparations are of limited concern, as plasma levels are low, and the intrauterine levels are much higher, so levels used intravaginally are often lower. Shaaban studied the effect of an intravaginal progesterone ring(10 mg/d) in 120 women and found no changes in growth and development of the infant or breastfeeding performance of the study participants. The author suggests the ring adds a measure of safety because the amount of steroid present in milk would be effectively absorbed from the infant's gut. Another new study also suggests no impact on breastfeeding following use of the intravaginal ring.

PROMETHAZINE; *Phenergan, Promethegan, Histanil, PMS Promethazine*	L2
Uses: Phenothiazine used as antihistamine	C

AAP: Not reviewed

T½= 12.7 hours; **RID**= ; **Oral** = 25%; **MW**= 284

Clinical: We have no data are available on the transfer of promethazine into breast milk, although it has been used clinically in pediatrics with no untoward effects. Observe for sedation and apnea. Ask about susceptibility of the infant to apnea. Some reports of promethazine linked to SIDS. Suitable alternative is diphenhydramine. There are numerous suggestions that his product may increase the risk of SIDS. Do not use in infants subject to apnea. Long term followup (6 years) has found no untoward effects on development.

PROPAFENONE; *Rythmol*	L2
Uses: Antiarrhythmic agent	C

AAP: Not reviewed

T½= 2-10 hours; **RID=** 0.09%; **Oral =** 12%; **MW=**

Clinical: Propafenone is a class 1C antiarrhythmic agent with structural similarities to propranolol. In one study the authors estimate that the daily intake of drug and active metabolite in their infant (3.3 kg) would have been 16 µg and 24 µg per day respectively.

PROPOFOL; *Diprivan*	L2
Uses: Preanesthetic sedative	B

AAP: Not reviewed

T½= 1-3 days; **RID=** 4.4%; **Oral =** ; **MW=** 178

Clinical: Minimal amounts of propofol are secreted into human milk with no untoward effects on the breastfed infant. Observe for sedation. Caution is advised in infant that have a history of apnea. One time usage is probably safe in breastfeeding. From the data currently available, it is apparent that only minimal amounts of propofol are transferred to human milk. No data are available on the oral absorption of propofol. Propofol is rapidly cleared from the neonatal circulation.

PROPOXYPHENE; *Darvocet N, Propacet, Darvon, Darvon-N, Novo-Propoxyn*	L2
Uses: Mild narcotic analgesic	C

AAP: Maternal medication usually compatible with breastfeeding

T½= 6-12 hours (propoxyphene); **RID=** ; **Oral =** Complete; **MW=** 339

Clinical: Propoxyphene is a mild narcotic analgesic similar in efficacy to aspirin. The amount secreted into milk is extremely low and is generally too low to produce effects in infant (<1 mg/day). Maternal plasma levels peak at 2 hours. Propoxyphene is metabolized to norpropoxyphene (which has weaker CNS effects). Adult half-life= 6-12 hours (propoxyphene), 30-36 hours (norpropoxyphene). The milk to plasma ratio averages 0.417 for propoxyphene, and 0.382 for norpropoxyphene. Thus far, no reports of untoward effects in infants have been reported.

PROPRANOLOL; *Inderal, Detensol, Novo-Pranol*	L2
Uses: Beta-blocker, antihypertensive	C

AAP: Maternal medication usually compatible with breastfeeding

$T\frac{1}{2}$= 3-5 hours; **RID**= 0.3% - 0.5%; **Oral** = 30%; **MW**= 259

Clinical: Propranolol is the preferred beta blocker for use in breastfeeding women since levels in milk are minimal. Use with caution in patients with asthma. Observe for bradycardia, sedation, hypotension in the breastfed infant. Long term exposure has not been studied, and caution is urged. Of the beta blocker family, propranolol is probably preferred in lactating women. Use with great caution, if at all, in mothers or infants with asthma.

PROPYLHEXEDRINE; *Benzedrex, Eventyl, Eventin*	L3
Uses: Decongestant	C

AAP: Not reviewed

$T\frac{1}{2}$= ; **RID**= ; **Oral** = ; **MW**= 155.3

Clinical: There are no adequate and well-controlled studies or case reports in breast feeding women

PROPYLTHIOURACIL; *PTU, Propyl-Thyracil*	L2
Uses: Antithyroid	D

AAP: Maternal medication usually compatible with breastfeeding

$T\frac{1}{2}$= 1-2 hours; **RID**= 1.8%; **Oral** = 50-95%; **MW**= 170

Clinical: Propylthiouracil is the preferred antithyroid agent in breastfeeding mothers. Only small amounts are secreted into milk, and side effects to the infant are minimal. To be safe, monitor thyroid function of the infant. No changes in infant thyroid have been reported. Monitor infant thyroid function (T4, TSH) carefully during therapy. See methimazole for a suitable alternative.

PSEUDOEPHEDRINE; *Sudafed, Halofed, Novafed, Eltor, Pseudofrin, Balminil, Contac*	**L3**
Uses: Decongestant	**C**
AAP: Maternal medication usually compatible with breastfeeding	
T½= <4 hours; **RID=** 4.7%; **Oral** = 90%; **MW=** 165	

Clinical: Pseudoephedrine is probably safe for use during breastfeeding. The problem is that pseudoephedrine usage during breastfeeding is linked to decreased milk production. Mothers with low milk supply should use caution or avoid pseudoephedrine usage for awhile. Observe for irritation in the breastfed infant. Therefore breastfeeding mothers with poor or marginal milk production should be exceedingly cautious in using pseudoephedrine. While there are anecdotal reports of its use in mothers with engorgement, we do not know if it is effective, or recommend its use for this purpose at this time.

PYRANTEL; *Pin-Rid, Reeses Pinworm, Antiminth, Pin-X, Combantrin*	**L3**
Uses: Anthelmintic	**C**
AAP: Not reviewed	
T½= ; **RID=** ; **Oral** = <50%; **MW=** 206	

Clinical: Pyrantel is an anthelmintic used to treat pinworm, hookworm, and round worm infestations. It is only minimally absorbed orally, with the majority being eliminated in feces. Peak plasma levels are generally less than 0.05 to 0.13 µg/mL and occur prior to 3 hours. Reported side effects are few and minimal. No data on transfer of pyrantel in human milk are available, but due to minimal oral absorption, and low plasma levels, it is unlikely that breastmilk levels would be clinically relevant. Generally it is administered as a single dose.

PYRAZINAMIDE; *Pyrazinamide, D-50, MK-56, PMS-pyrazinamide, Tebrazid*	**L3**
Uses: Antitubercular antibiotic	**C**

AAP: Not reviewed	

T½= 9-10 hours; **RID**= 1.5%; **Oral** = Complete; **MW**= 123

Clinical: Pyrazinamide is a typical antituberculosis antibiotic used as first-line therapy in tuberculosis infections. In one patient three hours following an oral dose of 1000 mg, peak milk levels were 1.5 mg/Liter of milk. Peak maternal plasma levels at 2 hours were 42 µg/mL.

PYRIDOSTIGMINE; *Mestinon, Regonol*	L2
Uses: Anticholinesterase muscle stimulant	C
AAP: Maternal medication usually compatible with breastfeeding	

T½= 3.3 hours; **RID**= 0.09%; **Oral** = 10-20%; **MW**= 261

Clinical: Pyridostigmine is a potent cholinesterase inhibitor used in myasthenia gravis to stimulate muscle strength. In a group of 2 mothers receiving from 120-300 mg/day, breastmilk concentrations varied from 5 to 25 µg/Liter. The calculated milk/plasma ratios varied from 0.36 to 1.13. No cholinergic side effects were noted and no pyridostigmine was found in the infants' plasma. Because the oral bioavailability is so poor (10-20%), the actual dose received by the breastfed infant would be significantly less than the above concentrations. Please note the dosage is highly variable and may be as high as 600 mg/day in divided doses. The authors estimated total daily intake at 0.1% or less of the maternal dose.

PYRIDOXINE; *Vitamin B-6, Hexa-Betalin*	L2
Uses: Vitamin B-6	A
AAP: Maternal medication usually compatible with breastfeeding	

T½= 15-20 days; **RID**= ; **Oral** = Complete; **MW**= 205

Clinical: Pyridoxine is vitamin B-6. The recommended daily allowance for non-pregnant women is 1.6 mg/day. Pyridoxine is secreted in milk in direct proportion to the maternal intake and concentrations in milk vary from 123 to 314 ng/mL depending on the study. Pyridoxine is required in slight excess during pregnancy and lactation and most prenatal vitamin supplements contain from 12-25 mg/day. Very high doses (600 mg/day) were reported to suppress prolactin secretion and therefore production of breastmilk. However, this data has been refuted in two studies where high doses of pyridoxine failed to suppress prolactin levels or lactation. It is not advisable to use in excess of 40 mg/day. One study clearly indicates that pyridoxine readily transfers into breastmilk and that B-6 levels in milk correlate closely with maternal intake, thus the reason for not using excessive doses. Breastfeeding mothers who are deficient in pyridoxine should be supplemented with modest amounts (<=40 mg/day).

PYRILAMINE; *Corzall, Dextrophenylpril, Polyhist*	L3
Uses: Anti-histamine	C
AAP: Not reviewed	
T½= ; RID= ; Oral = ; MW=	
Clinical: Pyrilamine is an antihistamine used in over-the-counter products. Like all other antihistamines, it may induce sedation. Suitable alternatives include: loratadine, cetirizine, or fexofenadine.	

PYRIMETHAMINE; *Daraprim*	L3
Uses: Antimalarial, folic acid antagonist	C
AAP: Maternal medication usually compatible with breastfeeding	
T½= 96 hours; RID= 45.8%; Oral = Complete; MW= 249	
Clinical: Pyrimethamine is a folic acid antagonist that has been used for prophylaxis of malaria. Maternal peak plasma levels occur 2-6 hours post-dose. Pyrimethamine is secreted into human milk. Milk levels ranged from 0.125 to 0.155 µg/L twenty four hours following the dose. An infant would receive an estimated dose of 3-4 mg in a 48 hour period (following 75 mg maternal dose). No adverse effects were reported in any of the infants.	

QUADRIVALENT HUMAN PAPILLMOAVIRUS VACCINE; *Gardasil*	L3
Uses: HPV vaccine	B

AAP: Not reviewed

T½= ; RID= ; Oral = ; MW=

Clinical: This is a non-infectious recombinant vaccine prepared from the purified virus like particles from the major capsid protein of four different virus types (6,11,16, and 18). Current recommendations are to begin the series in 11-26 year old females, with 4 weeks between the first and second doses, and 12 weeks between the second and third doses. It is not known whether vaccine antigens or antibodies are excreted in human milk. One study showed an increase risk of serious adverse event, but was judged by the investigator to be non-vaccine related. Also, a higher number of infants whose mothers received the vaccine had acute respiratory illnesses within 30 days after the vaccination.

QUAZEPAM; *Doral, Dormalin*	L2
Uses: Sedative, hypnotic	X

AAP: Drugs whose effect on nursing infants is unknown but may be of concern

T½= 39 hours; RID= 1.4%; Oral = Complete; MW= 387

Clinical: Quazepam is a long half-life benzodiazepine (Valium-like) medication used as a sedative and hypnotic. Including metabolites, one group of authors suggest that 17.1 μg of quazepam equivalents or 0.11% of the administered dose was recovered in milk. The authors estimated that 28.7 μg quazepam equivalents, or 0.19% of the quazepam dose would be excreted in breast milk every 24 hours.

QUETIAPINE FUMARATE; *Seroquel, Seroquel XR*	L2
Uses: Antipsychotic drug	C

AAP: Not reviewed

T½= 6 hours; RID= 0.07% - 0.1%; Oral = 100%; MW= 883

Clinical: New data suggests this neuroleptic drug penetrates milk poorly at a minimal dose of 200 mg/day. The RID would probably be < 0.43%. No untoward effects were noted in the infant. However, this will be a function of maternal dose. No adverse effects were reported in the infants in one study, but the authors suggest monitoring the infant's progress and quetiapine serum concentration.

QUINACRINE; *Atabrine*	L4
Uses: Antimalarial, giardiasis	C
AAP: Not reviewed	
T½= >5 days; **RID=** ; **Oral** = Complete; **MW=** 400	

Clinical: Quinacrine was once used for malaria but has been replaced by other preparations. It is primarily used for giardiasis. Small to trace amounts are secreted into milk. No known harmful effects except in infants with G6PD deficiencies. However, quinacrine is eliminated from the body very slowly, requiring up to 2 months for complete elimination. Quinacrine levels in liver are extremely high. Accumulation in infant is likely due to slow rate of excretion. Caution is urged.

QUINAPRIL; *Accupril, Accuretic*	L2
Uses: ACE inhibitor, antihypertensive	C
AAP: Not reviewed	
T½= 2 hours; **RID=** 1.6%; **Oral** = Complete; **MW=** 474	

Clinical: Quinapril is an angiotensin converting enzyme inhibitor (ACE) used as an antihypertensive. Accuretic products also contain the diuretic hydrochlorothiazide. In one study, levels of the active metabolite were not found in milk. The authors suggest that quinapril appears to be 'safe' during breastfeeding although, as always, the risk:benefit ratio should be considered when it is to be given to a nursing mother.

QUINIDINE; *Quinaglute, Quinidex, Apo-Quinidine, Cardioquin, Novo-Quinidin*	L2
Uses: Antiarrhythmic agent	C
AAP: Maternal medication usually compatible with breastfeeding	
T½= 6-8 hours; **RID=** 14.4%; **Oral** = 80%; **MW=** 324	

Clinical: Quinidine is used to treat cardiac arrhythmias. Three hours following a dose of 600 mg, the level of quinidine in the maternal serum was 9.0 mg/L and the concentration in her breast milk was 6.4 mg/L. Subsequently, a level of 8.2 mg/L was noted in breastmilk. Quinidine is selectively stored in the liver. Long-term use could expose an infant to liver toxicity. Monitor liver enzymes.

QUININE; *Quinamm, Novo-Quinine*	L2
Uses: Antimalarial	D

AAP: Maternal medication usually compatible with breastfeeding

T½= 11 hours; **RID**= 0.7% - 1.3%; **Oral** = 76%; **MW**= 324

Clinical: Quinine is a cinchona alkaloid primarily used in malaria prophylaxis and treatment. Small to trace amounts are secreted into milk. No reported harmful effects. In several studies, the total daily consumption by a breastfed infant was estimated to be 1-3 mg/day.

QUINUPRISTIN AND DALFOPRISTIN; *Synercid*	L3
Uses: Antimicrobial	B

AAP: Not reviewed

T½= 1-3 hours; **RID**= ; **Oral** = Nil; **MW**= 1022

Clinical: Synercid is a streptogramin antibacterial agent for intravenous use only. It is indicated for the treatment of vancomycin-resistant enterococcus faecium as well as for treatment of susceptible staph aureus. It has some use against methicillin-resistant organisms. No data are available on its transfer to human milk. However, due to its acidity and large molecular weight, milk levels will probably be low.

RABEPRAZOLE; *Aciphex*	L3
Uses: Antisecretory, antacid	B

AAP: Not reviewed

T½= 1-2 hours; **RID**= ; **Oral** = 52% (enteric); **MW**= 381

Clinical: We do not have any data on rabeprazole transfer into milk. Oral absorption is low and so absorption in the breastfed infant is probably minimal. Decreased stomach acidity may be a possible adverse effect. A suitable alternative is omeprazole. As presented in milk, it would be virtually destroyed in the infants stomach prior to absorption.

RABIES INFECTION; *Rabies Infection*	**L3**

Uses: Viral infection	

AAP: Not reviewed

T½= ; RID= ; Oral = ; MW=

Clinical: Rabies is an acute rapidly progressing illness caused by an RNA-containing virus that is usually fatal. Infection is via other warm-blooded mammals. Incubation is prolonged and can be up to 4-6 weeks. The virus multiplies locally, passes into local neurons and progressively ascends to the central nervous system. The virus is seldom found in the plasma compartment. The issue of breastfeeding following exposure to an animal bite is contentious and somewhat obscure. Person to person transmission has not been documented, nor has there been documentation of transmission of the rabies virus into human milk. If a breastfeeding women is exposed to the rabies virus, she should receive the human rabies immune globulin and begin the vaccination series. Most sources agree that once immunization has begun, the mother can continue breastfeeding. For a thorough review, see reference 4.

RABIES VACCINE; *Imovax Rabies Vaccine*	**L3**

Uses: Vaccination for rabies	C

AAP: Not reviewed

T½= ; RID= ; Oral = ; MW=

Clinical: Rabies vaccine is prepared from inactivated rabies virus. No data are available on transmission to breastmilk. Even if transferred to breastmilk, it is unlikely to produce untoward effects.

RADIOPAQUE AGENTS; *Omnipaque, Conray, Cholebrine, Telepaque, Oragrafin, Bilivist, Hypaque, Optiray*	**L2**

Uses: Radio-contrast agents	

AAP: Some approved by the American Academy of Pediatrics for use in breastfeeding mothers

T½= 20-90 minutes; **RID=** ; **Oral** = Minimal; **MW=**

Clinical: Radiopaque agents are probably compatible with breastfeeding since they are rapidly cleared from the body. Commonly used in pediatric patients for diagnostics. Try to avoid exposure to iodinated products if possible. Oral bioavailability is minimal, and the radiopaque agents should be unabsorbed in the infant's GI tract. Of the minimal amount in milk, virtually none is bioavailable to the infant as these agents are largely unabsorbed orally. According to several manufacturers, less than 0.005% of the iodine is free. These contrast agents are in essence pharmacologically inert, not metabolized, unabsorbed, and are rapidly excreted by the kidney (80-90% with 24 hours).

RALOXIFENE HCL; *Evista*	L3
Uses: Selective estrogen receptor modulator	X

AAP: Not reviewed

T½= 27-32 hours; **RID=** ; **Oral** = 2%; **MW=** 510

Clinical: Raloxifene is a selective estrogen receptor modulator. It blocks such estrogen effects as those that lead to breast cancer and uterine cancer. In addition, it also prevents bone loss and improved lipid profiles. It is used to prevent osteoporosis in postmenopausal women. It is poorly absorbed orally (2%).

RAMELTEON; *Rozerem*	L3
Uses: Nonbenzodiazepine hypnotic	C

AAP: Not reviewed

T½= 1-2.6 hours; **RID=** ; **Oral** = 1.8%; **MW=** 259

Clinical: Milk levels will probably be quite low due to its kinetics. It is unlikely to cause problems in a breastfeeding infant, but we as yet do not have milk levels. There have been no studies of levels of ramelteon in human milk. However, probable small amount in milk would only be 1.8% bioavailable. It is unlikely to sedate an infant.

RAMIPRIL; *Altace*	L3
Uses: ACE inhibitor, antihypertensive	C

AAP: Not reviewed

T½= 13-17 hours; **RID**= 0.3%; **Oral** = 60%; **MW**= 417

Clinical: Ramipril is used in hypertension. ACE inhibitors can cause increased fetal and neonatal morbidity and should not be used in pregnant women. Ingestion of a single 10 mg oral dose produced an undetectable level in breastmilk. However, animal studies have indicated that ramiprilat is transferred into milk in concentrations about one-third of those found in serum, but animal studies (lactation) are always high and do not at all correlate with humans. Only 0.25% of the total dose is estimated to penetrate into milk.

RANIBIZUMAB; *Lucentis*	**L3**
Uses: Angiogenesis inhibitor	C

AAP: Not reviewed

T½= 9 days; **RID**= ; **Oral** = Nil; **MW**= 48,000

Clinical: Large immunoglobulin. Unlikely to be absorbed orally in an infant, and even more unlikely to enter milk after the first week postpartum. No data are available on the transfer of ranibizumab into the milk compartment, however, due to the large molecular weight, it is unlikely that this drug would pose a threat to a breastfeeding infant after the first week postpartum.

RANITIDINE; *Zantac, Apo-Ranitidine, Novo-Ranidine, Nu-Ranit*	**L2**
Uses: Reduces gastric acid secretion	B

AAP: Not reviewed

T½= 2-3 hours; **RID**= 1.3% - 4.6%; **Oral** = 50%; **MW**= 314

Clinical: Ranitidine is commonly used in pediatrics at much higher doses. Ranitidine seems to concentrate in milk, although not nearly as much as therapeutic doses and it is probably safe to use during breastfeeding. There are no adverse effects reported in breastfed infants. Decreased stomach acidity is a possible side effect. See nizatidine or famotidine for alternatives.

REMIFENTANIL; *Ultiva*	**L3**
Uses: Opioid analgesic	C

AAP: Not reviewed

T½= 10-20 minutes; **RID**= ; **Oral** = Poor; **MW**= 412

Clinical: Remifentanil is a new opioid analgesic similar in potency and use as fentanyl. Although remifentanil has been found in rodent milk, no data are available on its transfer into human milk. It is cleared for use in children >2 years of age. As an analog of fentanyl, breastmilk levels should be similar and probably exceedingly low. In addition, remifentanil metabolism is not dependent on liver function and should be exceedingly short even in neonates. Due to its kinetics and brief half-life and its poor oral bioavailability, it is unlikely this product will produce clinically relevant levels in human breastmilk.

REPAGLINIDE; *Prandin, Gluconorm*	L4
Uses: Antidiabetic agent	C
AAP: Not reviewed	
T½= 1 hour; **RID**= ; **Oral** = 56%; **MW**=	

Clinical: Repaglinide is a hypoglycemic agent that lowers blood glucose levels in Type 2 non-insulin dependent diabetics. No data are available on its transfer to human milk, but rodent studies suggest that it may transfer into milk and induce hypoglycemic and skeletal changes in young animals via milk. Unfortunately, no dosing regimens were mentioned in these studies, so it is not known if normal therapeutic doses would produce such changes in humans. At this point, we do not know if it is safe for use in breastfeeding patients. But if it is used, the infant should be closely monitored for hypoglycemia and should not be fed until at least several hours after the dose to reduce exposure.

RESERPINE; *Raudixin, Serpasil*	L4
Uses: Antihypertensive	C
AAP: Not reviewed	
T½= 50-100 hours; **RID**= ; **Oral** = 40%; **MW**= 609	

Clinical: Reserpine is an old and seldom used antihypertensive. Reserpine is known to be secreted into human milk although the levels are unreported. Increased respiratory tract secretions, severe nasal congestion, cyanosis, and loss of appetite can occur. Some reports suggest no observable effect but should use with extreme caution if at all. Because safer, more effective products are available, reserpine should be avoided in lactating patients.

RETAPAMULIN; *Altabax*	L3
Uses: Antibacterial	B

AAP: Not reviewed

T½= ; **RID=** ; **Oral =** ; **MW=** 517.8

Clinical: Safe topical antibiotic cream. Systemic levels are almost too low to be detectable. Milk levels although not available, would be low to nil.

RHO (D) IMMUNE GLOBULIN; *Rhogam, Gamulin RH, Hyprho-D, Mini-Gamulin RH*	L2
Uses: Immune globulin	C

AAP: Not reviewed

T½= 24 days; **RID=** ; **Oral =** None; **MW=**

Clinical: RHO(D) immune globulin is an immune globulin prepared from human plasma containing high concentrations of Rh antibodies. Only trace amounts of anti-Rh are present in colostrum and none in mature milk in women receiving large doses of Rh immune globulin. No untoward effects have been reported. Most immunoglobulins are destroyed in the gastric acidity of the newborn infant. Rh immune globulins are not contraindicated in breastfeeding mothers.

RIBAVIRIN + INTERFERON ALFA-2B; *Rebetron*	L4
Uses: Antivirals for Hepatitis C treatment	X

AAP: Not reviewed

T½= 298 hours; **RID=** ; **Oral =** ; **MW=**

Clinical: Rebetron is a combination product containing the antiviral Ribavirin and the immunomodulator drug called interferon alfa-2b. This new combination product is indicated for the long-term treatment of hepatitis C. Rebetron is extremely dangerous to a fetus and is extremely teratogenic at doses even ½0th of the above therapeutic doses. Pregnancy must be strictly avoided if this product is used in either the male or female partner. Due to the long half-life of this product, pregnancy should be avoided for at least 6 months following use. This product should be considered hazardous to a breastfed infant.

RIBAVIRIN; *Virazole, Rebetol*	L4
Uses: Antiviral agent	X

AAP: Not reviewed

T½= 298 hours (SS); **RID=** ; **Oral** = 44%; **MW**= 244

Clinical: No data are available on its transfer to human milk, but it is probably low and its oral bioavailability is low as well. However, ribavirin concentrates in peripheral tissues and in the red blood cells in high concentrations over time (Vd= 802). Its elimination half-life at steady state averages 298 hours, which reflects slow elimination from non-plasma compartments. Red cell concentrations on average are 60 fold higher than plasma levels and may account for the occasional hemolytic anemia. It is likely the acute exposure of a breastfed infant would produce minimal side effects. However, chronic exposure over 6-12 months may be more risky, so caution is recommended.

RIBOFLAVIN; *Vitamin B-2, Abdec*	L1
Uses: Vitamin B2	A

AAP: Maternal medication usually compatible with breastfeeding

T½= 14 hours; **RID=** ; **Oral** = Complete; **MW**= 376

Clinical: Riboflavin is a B complex vitamin, also called Vitamin B-2. Riboflavin is absorbed by the small intestine by a well established transport mechanism. It is easily saturable, so excessive levels are not absorbed. Riboflavin is transported into human milk in concentrations proportional to dietary intake but generally averaged 400 ng/mL. Maternal supplementation is permitted if dose is not excessive. No untoward effects have been reported.

RIFAMPIN; *Rifadin, Rimactane, Rofact*	L2
Uses: Antitubercular drug	C

AAP: Maternal medication usually compatible with breastfeeding

T½= 3.5 hours; **RID=** 5.3% - 11.5%; **Oral** = 90-95%; **MW**= 823

Clinical: Rifampin usage in breastfeeding is relatively safe. Rifampin is secreted into human milk, although there have been no reports of adverse effects in breastfed infants. Observe for diarrhea in the breastfed infant.

RIFAXIMIN; *Xifaxan*	L3
Uses: Non-systemic antibiotic for diarrhea	C

AAP: Not reviewed

T½= 5.85 hours; **RID=** ; **Oral** = <0.4%; **MW**= 785

Clinical: This product is an intestinal antibiotic that produces only minimal levels in the plasma compartment. Oral bioavailability is less than 0.4%. While we have no studies in milk, the plasma levels are so low that it would probably be undetectable in human milk.

RIMANTADINE HCL; *Flumadine*	L3
Uses: Antiviral, anti-influenza A	C
AAP: Not reviewed	

T½= 25.4 hours; **RID**= ; **Oral** = 92%; **MW**= 179

Clinical: Rimantadine is an antiviral agent primarily used for influenza A infections. It is concentrated in rodent milk. Levels in animal milk 2-3 hours after administration were approximately twice those of the maternal serum, suggesting a milk/plasma ratio of about two. The manufacturer alludes to toxic side effects but fails to state them. No side effects yet reported in breastfeeding infants. Rimantadine is, however, indicated for prophylaxis of influenza A in pediatric patients >1 year of age.

RISEDRONATE; *Actonel*	L3
Uses: Prevents bone resorption	C
AAP: Not reviewed	

T½= 480 hours; **RID**= ; **Oral** = 0.63%; **MW**= 305

Clinical: Risedronate is a bisphosphonate that slows the dissolution of hydroxyapatite crystals in the bone, thus reducing bone calcium loss in certain syndromes such as Paget's syndrome. Its penetration into milk is possible due to its small molecular weight, but it has not yet been reported except in rats. However, due to the presence of fat and calcium in milk, its oral bioavailability in infants would be exceedingly low. However, the presence of this product in an infant's growing bones is concerning, and due caution is recommended.

RISPERIDONE; *Risperdal, Invega*	L3
Uses: Antipsychotic	C
AAP: Not reviewed	

T½= 3-20 hours; **RID**= 2.8% - 9.1%; **Oral** = 70-94%; **MW**= 410

Clinical: Risperidone is probably okay to use in breastfeeding. No adverse effects have been reported in breastfeeding infants. Risperidone may increase milk production due to elevation of prolactin. Quetiapine may be a suitable alternative since there is less transfer into human milk.

RITODRINE; *Pre-Par, Yutopar*	L3
Uses: Adrenergic agent	B
AAP: Not reviewed	
T½= 15 hours; **RID**= ; **Oral** = 30%; **MW**= 287	

Clinical: Ritodrine is primarily used to reduce uterine contractions in premature labor due to its beta-2 adrenergic effect on uterine receptors. No data are available on its transfer to human milk.

RITONAVIR; *Norvir*	L3
Uses: Antiretroviral agent used in HIV infections.	B
AAP: Not reviewed	
T½= T ½ = 3-5 hrs; **RID**= ; **Oral** = undetermined; **MW**= 720.95	

Clinical: There are no adequate and well-controlled studies or case reports in breastfeeding women. Breastfeeding is not recommended in mothers who have HIV. No data are available on its tranfer into human milk.

RITUXIMAB; *Rituxan*	L3
Uses: Antineoplastic agent, monoclonal antibody	C
AAP: Not reviewed	
T½= 206 hours; **RID**= ; **Oral** = Nil; **MW**= 145,000	

Clinical: This is another IgG product that is unlikely to enter milk, nor be orally bioavailable in the infant. However, we do not have any reports of its use in breastfeeding mothers. There are no reported levels in human milk. Levels of IgG antibodies in human milk are generally low. In addition, oral bioavailability of this protein is likely to be nil.

RIZATRIPTAN; *Maxalt*	L3
Uses: Antimigraine	C
AAP: Not reviewed	
T½= 2-3 hours; **RID**= ; **Oral** = 45%; **MW**= 269	

Clinical: Rizatriptan is a selective serotonin receptor agonist, similar in effect to sumatriptan. It is primarily indicated for acute migraine headache treatment. No data are available on its transfer into human milk, but it is concentrated in rodent milk (M/P=5). Until we have clear data on breastmilk levels, the kinetics of this drug may predispose to higher milk levels and sumatriptan should be preferred. Wait 4 hrs after dose then may breastfeed.

ROPINIROLE; *Requip*	L4
Uses: Dopamine stimulating agent used for Restless Legs and Parkinson's syndrome	C

AAP: Not reviewed

T½= 6 hours; **RID=** ; **Oral** = 55%; **MW**= 297

Clinical: Ropinirole is a dopamine agonist and would likely reduce prolactin levels, hence reducing milk production. Use only as a last resort if at all. This product can induce hallucinations and immediate sleepiness similar to narcolepsy. High risk of nausea (60%) and dizziness(40%).

ROPIVACAINE; *Naropin*	L2
Uses: Local anesthetic	B

AAP: Not reviewed

T½= 4.2 hours (epidural); **RID=** ; **Oral** = ; **MW**= 328

Clinical: Ropivacaine is a newer local anesthetic commonly used as a regional anesthetic and for epidural infusions. It is believed to produce less hypotension when compared to bupivacaine. No data are available on its transfer into human milk, but the manufacture suggests it is probably much lower than the infant receives in utero. This agent is commonly used in obstetrics and probably poses few if any problems to a breastfeeding infant.

ROSIGLITAZONE; *Avandia*	L3
Uses: Oral antidiabetic agent	C

AAP: Not reviewed

T½= 3-4 hours; **RID=** ; **Oral** = 99%; **MW**= 357

Clinical: Rosiglitazone is an oral antidiabetic agent which acts primarily by increasing insulin sensitivity. In essence, the insulin receptor is activated reducing insulin resistance. It also decreases hepatic gluconeogenesis and increases insulin-dependent muscle glucose uptake. It does not increase the release of or secretion of insulin. No data are available on its entry into human milk. The maximum plasma concentration following a 2 mg dose is only 156 nanograms/mL. Assuming a dose of 2 mg every 12 hours and a theoretical milk/plasma ratio of 1.0 (which is probably high), an infant would likely ingest about 23.4 μg/kg/day via milk. In a 5 kg infant, this would be approximately 2.8% of the maternal dose. But these data are only theoretical.

ROSUVASTATIN CALCIUM; *Crestor*	L3
Uses: HMG-CoA reductase inhibitor	X

AAP: Not reviewed

T½= 19 hours; **RID=** ; **Oral =** 20%; **MW=** 1001

Clinical: Rosuvastatin, like other statins, is used to reduce cholesterol in patients with hypercholesterolemia. No data are available on the excretion of this product into human milk, however due to the large molecular weight and high protein binding, it would be unlikely that a therapeutic concentration would be passed to a breastfeeding infant. The use of anti-hyperlipidemia medications would not be advisable under most circumstances in breastfeeding mothers.

ROTIGOTINE; *Neupro*	L4
Uses: Dopamine agonist	C

AAP: Not reviewed

T½= 5-7 hours; **RID=** ; **Oral =** ; **MW=** 315.48

Clinical: Rotigotine is a dopamine agonist used to treat the signs and symptoms of Parkinson's disease. No data are available on the transfer of rotigotine into human milk. According to the manufacturer, rotigotine stimulates dopamine and thus reduces prolactin secretion from the pituitary. It is possible that this medication could significantly decrease prolactin release and in turn, decrease milk production. Therefore, milk production should be monitored carefully if this medication is used in a lactating mother.

RUBELLA VIRUS VACCINE, LIVE; *Meruvax,* *Rubella Vaccine, Measles Vaccine*	L2
Uses: Live attenuated (measles) vaccine	X

AAP: Not reviewed

T½= ; **RID=** ; **Oral =** ; **MW=**

Clinical: Rubella virus vaccine contains a live attenuated virus. The American College of Obstetricians and Gynecologists and the CDC currently recommends the early postpartum immunization of women who show no or low antibody titers to rubella. At least four studies have found rubella virus to be transferred via milk although presence of clinical symptoms was not evident. Rubella virus has been cultured from the throat of one infant while another infant was clinically ill with minor symptoms and serologic evidence of rubella infection. In general, the use of rubella virus vaccine in breastfeeding mothers of full-term, normal infants has not been associated with untoward effects and is generally recommended.

SACCHARIN; *Saccharin*	L3
Uses: Sweetener	C

AAP: Not reviewed

T½= 4.84 hours; **RID=** 3.6%; **Oral =** Complete; **MW=** 183

Clinical: In one group of 6 women who received 126 mg (per 12 oz drink) every 6 hours for 9 doses, milk levels varied greatly from <200 µg/L after one dose to 1.765 mg/L after 9 doses. Under these dosing conditions, saccharin levels appear to accumulate over time. Half-life in serum and milk were 4.84 hours and 17.9 hours respectively after 3 days. Even after such doses, these milk levels are considered minimal. Moderate intake should be compatible with nursing.

SAGE; *Sage, Dalmatian, Spanish*	L4
Uses: Herbal product	

AAP: Not reviewed

T½= ; **RID=** ; **Oral =** ; **MW=**

Clinical: Extracts and teas have been used to treat digestive disorders (antispasmodic), as an antiseptic and astringent, for treating diarrhea, gastritis, sore throat, and other maladies. The dried and smoked leaves have been used for treating asthma symptoms. Sage extracts have been found to be strong antioxidants and with some antimicrobial properties (staph. aureus) due to the phenolic acid salvin content. For the most part, sage is relatively nontoxic and nonirritating. Ingestion of significant quantities may lead to cheilitis, stomatitis, dry mouth, or local irritation. Due to drying properties and pediatric hypersensitivity to anticholinergics, sage should be used with some caution in breastfeeding mothers.

SALICYLIC ACID, TOPICAL; *Occlusal-HP*	L3

Uses: Keratolytic, Antiacne

AAP: Not reviewed

T½= ; RID= ; Oral = ; MW= 138.12

Clinical: Transcutaneous absorption is significant with these products. Avoid use in breastfeeding mothers. Salicylic acid is often used in anti-acne preparations, as well as in many wart and corn removal products. Systemic absorption depends on the concentration of the product used, the amount applied, and duration of use. Absorption increases with the duration of use. The systemic absorption relative to the dose has been found to range from 9.3 to 25.1%. Due to systemic absorption, topical salicylic acid should not be used while breastfeeding. It is known that salicylates are excreted in mothers' milk, and may possibly contribute to certain conditions such as Reye's syndrome in children.

SALMETEROL XINAFOATE; *Serevent*	L2
Uses: Long acting beta adrenergic bronchodilator	C

AAP: Not reviewed

T½= 5.5 hours; RID= ; Oral = Complete; MW=

Clinical: Salmeterol has minimal systemic absorption from the inhaled route of administration. Oral dosing has complete absorption and may transfer to human milk. Observe for tremors and excitement in the breastfed infant. No reports of use in lactating women are available.

SALSALATE; *Amigesic, Salflex*	L4
Uses: NSAID	C

AAP: Drugs associated with significant side effects and should be given with caution

T½= 7-8 hours; **RID=** ; **Oral =** Complete; **MW=** 258

Clinical: Salsalate is a non-steroidal anti-inflammatory drug used to treat minor pain or fever and arthritis. Salsalate is similar to salicylic acid, that when ingested releases pure salicylic acid. Absorption of salicylic acid (SA) is complete. SA inhibits prostaglandin synthesis and acts on the hypothalamus heat-regulating center to reduce fever. Salicylic acid is excreted in breast milk (see aspirin) and chronic use of salicylates should be avoided. Therefore, salsalate should probably not be used while breastfeeding.

SAQUINAVIR; *Fortovase, Invirase*	L4
Uses: Antiretroviral agent used in HIV infections	B

AAP: Not reviewed

T½= ; **RID=** ; **Oral =** 331 % (relative bioavailability); **MW=** 670.86

Clinical: There are no adequate and well-controlled studies or case reports in breastfeeding women. Breastfeeding is not recommended in mothers who have HIV. No studies on secretion of drug into milk.

SCOPOLAMINE; *Transderm Scope, Transderm-V, Buscopan*	L3
Uses: Anticholinergic	C

AAP: Maternal medication usually compatible with breastfeeding

T½= 2.9 hours; **RID=** ; **Oral =** 27%; **MW=** 303

Clinical: Scopolamine is a typical anticholinergic used primarily for motion sickness and preoperatively to produce amnesia and decrease salivation. There are no reports on its transfer into human milk, but due to its poor oral bioavailability it is generally believed to be minimal. However, following prolonged exposure in a newborn, some anticholinergic symptoms could appear, and include drying, constipation, and urinary retention.

SECOBARBITAL; *Seconal, Novo-Secobarb*	L3
Uses: Short acting barbiturate sedative	D

AAP: Maternal medication usually compatible with breastfeeding

$T\frac{1}{2}$= 15-40 hours; **RID**= ; **Oral** = 90%; **MW**= 260

Clinical: Secobarbital is a sedative, hypnotic barbiturate. It is probably secreted into breastmilk, although levels are unknown, and may be detectable in milk for 24 hours or longer. Recommend mothers delay breastfeeding for 3-4 hours to reduce possible transfer to infant if exposure to this barbiturate is required.

SELEGILINE; *Eldepryl, Emsam, Zelapar*	L4
Uses: Monoamine Oxidase Inhibitor	C

AAP: Not reviewed

$T\frac{1}{2}$= 10 hours; **RID**= ; **Oral** = 5.5%; **MW**= 187

Clinical: This is a typical and irreversible MAO inhibitor. This product has numerous and severe drug-drug interactions and drug-food interactions. MAO inhibitors are too hazardous to be used in breastfeeding mothers. This product should not be used in breastfeeding mothers.

SELENIUM SULFIDE; *Selsun, Exsel, Head and Shoulders, Selsun Blue*	L3
Uses: Topical antimicrobial	

AAP: Not reviewed

$T\frac{1}{2}$= ; **RID**= ; **Oral** = ; **MW**=

Clinical: Selenium sulfide is an anti-infective compound with mild antibacterial and antifungal activity. It is commonly used for Tinea Versicolor and seborrheic dermatitis such as dandruff. Selenium is not apparently absorbed significantly through intact skin but is absorbed by damaged skin or open lesions. There are no data on its transfer into human milk. If used properly on undamaged skin, it is very unlikely that enough would be absorbed systemically to produce untoward effects in a breastfed infant. Do not apply directly to nipple as enhanced absorption by the infant could occur.

SENNA LAXATIVES; *Senokot, Senexon, Ex Lax, Senna-Gen, Black-Draught, Fletcher's Castoria, Agoral*

L3

Uses: Laxative

AAP: Maternal medication usually compatible with breastfeeding

T½= ; **RID=** ; **Oral =** ; **MW=**

Clinical: Short-term usage of senna during breastfeeding is probably okay. Transfer of senna into milk appears to be low, although this is not confirmed. In one study of 23 women who received Senokot (100 mg containing 8.602 mg of Sennosides A and B), no sennoside A or B was detectable in their milk. Of 15 mothers reporting loose stools, two infants had loose stools. Observe for loose stools in the breastfed infant. Advise patient about increasing dietary fiber intake and a regular exercise regimen. PEG laxatives (Miralax) is a suitable alternative since it is safe and efficacious.

SERTRALINE; *Zoloft*

L2

Uses: Antidepressant

C

AAP: Drugs whose effect on nursing infants is unknown but may be of concern

T½= 26 hours; **RID=** 0.4% - 2.2%; **Oral =** Complete; **MW=** 306

Clinical: Sertraline has been extensively studied in many breastfeeding mothers. The data is consistent that levels in milk are quite low and do not normally affect an infant. Studies of platelet function further suggest that sertraline is poorly absorbed by the infant and at levels too low to affect platelet function. Sertraline is a preferred antidepressant.

SEVOFLURANE; *Ultane*

L3

Uses: Anesthetic gas

B

AAP: Not reviewed

T½= 1.8-3.8 hours; **RID=** ; **Oral =** ; **MW=** 200

Clinical: Sevoflurane is a gaseous halogenated general anesthetic drug that is particularly popular because of its rapid wash-out. Average patient time to emergence is approximately 8.2 minutes. It is commonly used in adult and pediatric patients, and is used in cesarean sections. The manufacturer states that while the concentration of sevoflurane have not been measured in breastmilk, they are probably of no clinical importance 24 hours after anesthesia. Because of its rapid wash-out, sevoflurane concentrations in milk are predicted to be below those found with many other volatile anesthatics. While no data on levels of sevoflurane in breast milk are available, this product, due to its rapid clearance from the body (100 fold drop in 120 minutes), should not pose a problem for continued breastfeeding soon after exposure.

SIBUTRAMINE; *Meridia*	L4
Uses: Appetite suppressant	C
AAP: Not reviewed	
T½= 12.5-21.8 hours; **RID=** ; **Oral** = 77%; **MW**= 334	

Clinical: Sibutramine is a nonamphetamine appetite suppressant. Due to its effect on serotonin and norepinephrine reuptake, it is considered an antidepressant as well. Sibutramine is rather small in molecular weight, active in the CNS, extremely lipid soluble, and has two 'active' metabolites with long half-lives (14-16 hours). Although no data are available on its transfer into human milk, the pharmacokinetics of this drug theoretically suggest that it might have a rather high milk/plasma ratio and could enter milk in significant levels. Until we know more, a risk assessment may not support the use of this product in breastfeeding mothers.

SILDENAFIL; *Viagra, Revatio*	L3
Uses: For erectile dysfunction and pulmonary hypertension	B
AAP: Not reviewed	
T½= 4 hours; **RID=** ; **Oral** = 40%; **MW**= 666	

Clinical: Sildenafil is an inhibitor of nitrous oxide metabolism, thus increasing levels of nitrous oxide, smooth muscle relaxation, and an increased flow of blood in the corpus cavernosum of the penis. While not currently indicated for women, illicit use is increasing. No data are available on the transfer of sildenafil into human milk, but it is unlikely that significant transfer will occur due to its larger molecular weight and short half-life. However, caution is recommended in breastfeeding mothers. While not reported, persistent abnormal erections (priapism) could potentially occur in male infants.

SILICONE BREAST IMPLANTS	L3

Uses: Silicone mammoplasty

AAP: Not reviewed

T½= ; **RID=** ; **Oral =** ; **MW=**

Clinical: Silicone transfer to breastmilk has been studied in one group of 15 lactating mothers with bilateral silicone breast implants. Silicon levels were measured in breastmilk, whole blood, cow's milk, and 26 brands of infant formula. Comparing implanted women to controls, mean silicon levels were not significantly different in breastmilk or in blood. Mean silicon level measured in store-bought cow's milk was high. The authors concluded that lactating women with silicone implants are similar to control women with respect to levels of silicon in their breastmilk and blood. From these studies, silicon levels are 10 times higher in cow's milk and even higher in infant formulas.

SILVER SULFADIAZINE; *Silvadene, SSD Cream, Thermazene, Flamazine, Dermazin, SSD*	L3
Uses: Topical antimicrobial cream	B

AAP: Not reviewed

T½= 10 hours (sulfa); **RID=** ; **Oral =** Complete; **MW=**

Clinical: Silver sulfadiazine is a topical antimicrobial cream primarily used for reducing sepsis in burn patients. The silver component is not absorbed from the skin. Sulfadiazine is partially absorbed. After prolonged therapy of large areas, sulfadiazine levels in plasma may approach therapeutic levels. Although sulfonamides are known to be secreted into human milk, they are not particularly problematic except in the newborn period when they may produce kernicterus.

SIMETHICONE	L3

Uses: OTC active ingredient

AAP: Not reviewed

T½= ; **RID=** ; **Oral =** ; **MW=**

Clinical: Because the drug is not absorbed, the risk to a nursing infant from maternal use of simethicone is thought to be negligible. There was no evidence of medication-related adverse effects in the neonate with simethicone exposure.

SIMVASTATIN; *Zocor*	L3

Uses: Reduces cholesterol   X

AAP: Not reviewed

T½= Long; **RID=** ; **Oral =** Poor; **MW=** 419

Clinical: Simvastatin reduces blood cholesterol levels. Others in this family are known to be secreted into human and rodent milk, but no data are available on simvastatin. It is likely that milk levels will be low because less than 5% of simvastatin reaches the plasma, most being removed first-pass by the liver.

SINCALIDE; *Kinevac*	L3

Uses: Diagnostic agent for cholecystography   B

AAP: Not reviewed

T½= Brief; **RID=** ; **Oral =** Nil; **MW=** 1143

Clinical: Kinevac is a synthetic, C-terminal octapeptide fragment of cholecystokinin, a cystopancreatic-gastrointestinal hormone peptide which when injected produces a substantial contracture of the gall bladder. Sincalide is therefore used to assess biliary and gall bladder function. No data are available on the transfer of this peptide into human milk, but due to its molecular weight it is extremely unlikely significant quantities would ever reach the milk compartment. It has a brief but unreported half-life.

SIROLIMUS; *Rapamune, Rapamycin, NSC-226080*	L4

Uses: Immunosuppressant   C

AAP: Not reviewed

T½= 57-63 hours; **RID=** ; **Oral =** 15%; **MW=** 914

Clinical: Sirolimus is an immunosuppressant sometimes used in combination with cyclosporin in renal transplants. No data are available on its transfer to human milk. Average plasma levels are quite low (264 ng x hr/mL) and the drug is strongly attached to cellular components and plasma levels are low. It is not likely it will penetrate milk in levels that are significant. However, it is a potent inhibitor of the enzyme 70 K S6 kinase, which is stimulated in breast tissue by prolactin. This agent, in rodent mammary tissue, strongly inhibits milk component production. It could potentially suppress milk production in lactating mothers and caution is recommended.

SITAGLIPTIN PHOSPHATE; *Januvia*	L3
Uses: Antidiabetic agent in Type 2 diabetics	B

AAP: Not reviewed

T½= 12 hours; **RID=** ; **Oral =** 87%; **MW=** 523

Clinical: It is unlikely that this product when finally studied will produce significant levels in human milk. However at this point one should be cautious. It does not product hypoglycemia in healthy, nondiabetic individuals, so its use in a breastfeeding mother is unlikely to bother an infant. But caution is still recommended.

SODIUM OXYBATE; *Xyrem*	L4
Uses: CNS depressant	B

AAP: Not reviewed

T½= 0.5-1 hour; **RID=** ; **Oral =** 25%; **MW=** 126

Clinical: This sedative is likely to enter milk significantly and should be used only very cautiously in a breastfeeding mother. Sodium oxybate is a central nervous system depressant used to treat excessive daytime sleepiness and cataplexy in patients with narcolepsy. Its mechanism of action is unknown, but it may work by inhibiting GABA receptors. No data are available on the transfer of oxybate into human breastmilk, but due to the low molecular weight and low protein binding, it is likely this medication will be secreted in human milk and be passed to a breastfeeding infant. Due to the sedative properties of this drug, this product should be used very cautiously in breastfeeding mothers, if at all.

SODIUM TETRADECYL SULFATE; *Sotradecol*	L3

Uses: Sclerosing Agent

AAP: Not reviewed

T½= ; **RID=** ; **Oral =** ; **MW=** 316

Clinical: Sodium tetradecyl sulfate (STS) is a sclerosing agent used to treat varicose veins. There are no data available on its transfer into human milk. There are no studies done in nursing women.

SOLIFENACIN SUCCINATE; *VESIcare*	L4
Uses: Muscarinic agonist for bladder hyperactivity	C

AAP: Not reviewed

T½= 45-68 hours; **RID=** ; **Oral =** 90%; **MW=** 480

Clinical: Solifenacin is a potent anticholinergic. Its structure is much larger than that of atropine and would probably limit its transfer to milk, but at present we don't have milk levels. Unfortunately, its half-life in adults approaches 68 hours. Should the clinician decide that the need is great, and the mother insists on breastfeeding, then observe the infant for urinary retention, and other anticholinergic symptoms. In reality, I think these symptoms are probably unlikely.

SOMATREM, SOMATROPIN; *Human Growth Hormone, Nutropin, Humatrope, Growth Hormone, Saizen, Norditropin, Protropin*	L3
Uses: Human growth hormone	C

AAP: Not reviewed

T½= ; **RID=** ; **Oral =** Poor; **MW=** 22,124

Clinical: Somatrem and somatropin are purified polypeptide hormones of recombinant DNA origin. It is a large protein. They are structurally similar or identical to human growth hormone (hGH). One study in 16 women indicates that hGH treatment for 7 days stimulated breastmilk production by 18.5% (verses 11.6% in controls) in a group of normal lactating women. No adverse effects were noted. Leukemia has occurred in a small number of children receiving hGH, but the relationship is uncertain. Because it is a peptide of 191 amino acids and its molecular weight is so large, its transfer into milk is very unlikely. Further, its oral absorption would be minimal to nil.

SOTALOL; *Betapace, Sotacor, Apo-Sotalol, Rylosol*	L3
Uses: Antihypertensive, beta-blocker	B
AAP: Maternal medication usually compatible with breastfeeding	

T½= 12 hours; **RID=** 25.5%; **Oral** = 90-100%; **MW=** 272

Clinical: Sotalol is a typical beta blocker antihypertensive with low lipid solubility. It is secreted into milk in high levels. Sotalol concentrations in milk ranged from 4.8 to 20.2 mg/L (mean= 10.5 mg/L) in 5 mothers. Although these milk levels appear high, no evidence of toxicity was noted in 12 infants. It is suggested that if a mother decides to breastfeed while taking sotalol, the baby should receive close monitoring for side effects.

SPIRONOLACTONE; *Aldactone, Novospiroton*	L2
Uses: Potassium sparing diuretic	D
AAP: Maternal medication usually compatible with breastfeeding	

T½= 10-35 hours; **RID=** 4.3%; **Oral** = 70%; **MW=** 417

Clinical: Spironolactone is metabolized to canrenone, which is known to be secreted into breastmilk. Milk levels reported in several studies are low.

ST. JOHN'S WORT; *St. John's Wort, Saint John's Wort, SJW*	L2
Uses: Antidepressant	
AAP: Not reviewed	

T½= 26.5 hours; **RID=** ; **Oral** = ; **MW=** 504

Clinical: Breastfeeding studies are rather weak, but suggest minimal transfer of SJW into human milk. This product is probably safe to use in breastfeeding mothers. However, the drug-drug interactions are major. SJW stimulates liver y drug metabolism, and has been reported to reduce varius drug plasma levels by 50% or more.   Do not use while taking other important drugs (birth control, anticonvulsant, antihypertensiver, etc).

STREPTOMYCIN	L3
Uses: Antibiotic	D
AAP: Maternal medication usually compatible with breastfeeding	

T½= 2.6 hours; **RID=** 0.3% - 0.6%; **Oral** = Poor; **MW=** 582

Clinical: Streptomycin is an aminoglycoside antibiotic from the same family as gentamicin. It is primarily administered IM or IV although it is seldom used today with exception of the treatment of tuberculosis. Because the oral absorption of streptomycin is very poor, absorption by infant is probably minimal (unless premature or early neonate).

STRONTIUM-89 CHLORIDE; *Metastron*	L5
Uses: Radioactive product for bone pain	D

AAP: Not reviewed

$T\frac{1}{2}$= 50.5 days; **RID**= ; **Oral** = ; **MW**= 159

Clinical: Metastron behaves similarly to calcium. It is rapidly cleared from plasma and sequestered into bone where its radioactive emissions relieve metastatic bone pain. Radioactive half-life is 50.5 days. Transfer into milk is unreported but likely. This radioactive product is too dangerous to use in lactating mothers.

SUCCIMER; *Chemet*	L3
Uses: Lead Chelator for lead poisoning	C

AAP: Not reviewed

$T\frac{1}{2}$= 2 -48 hours; **RID**= ; **Oral** = Complete; **MW**= 182

Clinical: Succimer is a chelating agent containing dimercaptosuccinic acid. It is commonly used to chelate and increase the urinary excretion of lead. While removing lead is important, some chelators (EDTA) are noted for increasing the plasma levels of lead and promoting its migration to neural and other tissues. In the instance of a breastfeeding woman, this could theoretically increase milk lead levels. However, succimer as studied in rodents has been found to increase the urinary elimination of lead without redistribution of lead to other compartments (this would theoretically include milk). While we do not have studies of succimer transfer into human milk, due to its low pKa of succimer, it is unlikely that lead, chelated to succimer, would transfer into human milk. But this is not known for sure. If breastfeeding patients were to pump and discard milk for 5 days while under therapy with succimer, it would significantly remove the risk of lead transfer into milk (if this occurs). However, more data are required before breastfeeding can be recommended following the use of succimer.

SUCRALFATE; *Carafate, Sulcrate, Novo-Sucralfate, Nu-Sucralfate*	L2
Uses: For peptic ulcers	B
AAP: Not reviewed	
T½= ; **RID=** ; **Oral =** <5%; **MW=** 2087	
Clinical: Sucralfate is a sucrose aluminum complex used for stomach ulcers. When administered orally sucralfate forms a complex that physically covers stomach ulcers. Less than 5% is absorbed orally. At these plasma levels it is very unlikely to penetrate into breastmilk.	

SUCRALOSE; *Splenda*	L1
Uses: Sweetener	
AAP: Not reviewed	
T½= ; **RID=** ; **Oral =** ; **MW=**	
Clinical: There are no adequate or well-controlled case reports in breastfeeding women. Sucralose is not fully absorbed, and is excreted unchanged in the urine; no toxicity or carcinogenic activity has been noted in animal studies. FDA deems sucralose is safe for consumption in pregnant and lactating women.	

SULCONAZOLE NITRATE; *Exelderm*	L3
Uses: Antifungal cream	C
AAP: Not reviewed	
T½= ; **RID=** ; **Oral =** ; **MW=**	
Clinical: Exelderm is a broad-spectrum antifungal topical cream. Although no data exist on transfer into human milk, it is unlikely that the degree of transdermal absorption would be high enough to produce significant milk levels. Only 8.7% of the topically administered dose is transcutaneously absorbed.	

SULFASALAZINE; *Azulfidine, PMS Sulfasalazine, Salazopyrin, SAS-500*	L3
Uses: Anti-inflammatory for ulcerative colitis	B
AAP: Drugs associated with significant side effects and should be given with caution	
T½= 7.6 hours; **RID=** 0.3% - 1.1%; **Oral =** Poor; **MW=** 398	

Clinical: 5-Aminosalicylic acid is poorly absorbed orally, so levels in milk are quite low as per all these studies. With exception of one report, this product appears quite safe for breastfeeding mothers and their infants. Few if any adverse effects have been observed in most nursing infants. However, one reported case of toxicity which may have been an idiosyncratic allergic response. Use with some caution caution, observing for watery stools, or diarrhea.

SULFISOXAZOLE; *Gantrisin, AZO-Gantrisin, Novo-Soxazole, Sulfizole*	**L2**
Uses: Sulfonamide antibiotic	**C**
AAP: Maternal medication usually compatible with breastfeeding	
T½= 4.6-7.8 hours; **RID**= ; **Oral** = 100%; **MW**= 267	

Clinical: Sulfisoxazole is a popular, sulfonamide antimicrobial. It is secreted in breastmilk in small amounts although the actual levels are somewhat controversial. In one study, less than 1% of the maternal dose was secreted into human milk. This is probably insufficient to produce problems in a normal newborn. Sulfisoxazole appears to be best choice with lowest milk/plasma ratio. Use with caution in weakened infants or those with hyperbilirubinemia.

SULPIRIDE	**L2**
Uses: Antidepressant, antipsychotic	
AAP: Not reviewed	
T½= 6-8 hours; **RID**= 2.7% - 20.7%; **Oral** = 27-34%; **MW**= 341	

Clinical: Sulpiride is a selective dopamine antagonist used as an antidepressant and antipsychotic. Sulpiride is a strong neuroleptic antipsychotic drug; however, several studies using smaller doses have found it to significantly increase prolactin levels and breastmilk production in smaller doses that do not produce overt neuroleptic effects on the mother. In two studies, no untoward effects were noted inbreastfed infants. The authors concluded that sulpiride, when administered early in the postpartum period, is useful in promoting initiation of lactation.

SUMATRIPTAN SUCCINATE; *Imitrex, Treximet, Alsuma, Sumavel DosePro*	**L3**
Uses: Anti-migraine medication	**C**
AAP: Maternal medication usually compatible with breastfeeding	

T½= 1.3 hours; **RID**= 3.5% - 15.3%; **Oral** = 10-15%; **MW**= 413

Clinical: Sumatriptan transfer into human milk appears to be minimal, although 15% of the maternal dose has been detected in milk which is considerably high. There are no reports of adverse effects in breastfed infants. Potential adverse effects to watch out for are flushing and dizziness.

SYNEPHRINE; *Bitter Orange, Advantra*	L4

Uses: Weight-loss agent

AAP: Not reviewed

T½= 2- 3 hours; **RID**= ; **Oral** = 22%; **MW**= 167

Clinical: Synephrine is commonly used as an ephedra-free weight loss agent. There is little to no data on its effects during lactation. It is likely transferred into breast milk due to its small size and large volume of distribution. Acute usage in breast-feeding mothers may have little harm; it is not advised for long-term usage.

TACROLIMUS; *Prograf, Protopic, Protopic*	L3
Uses: Immunosuppressant	C

AAP: Not reviewed

T½= 34.2 hours; **RID**= 0.1% - 0.5%; **Oral** = 14-32%; **MW**= 822

Clinical: Tacrolimus is an immunosuppressant. It is used to reduce rejection of transplanted organs including liver and kidney. In several studies the authors suggest that maternal therapy with tacrolimus for liver transplant may be compatible with breastfeeding. Recently the FDA has approved a topical form of tacrolimus (Protopic). Absorption via skin is minimal. Combined with the poor oral bioavailability of this product, it is not likely a breastfed infant will receive enough following topical use (maternal) to produce adverse effects.

TAMOXIFEN; *Nolvadex, Apo-Tamox, Tamofen, Tamone*	L5
Uses: Anti-estrogen, anticancer	D

AAP: Not reviewed

T½= >7 days; **RID**= ; **Oral** = Complete; **MW**= 371

Clinical: Tamoxifen is a nonsteroidal antiestrogen. It attaches to the estrogen receptor and produces only minimal stimulation, thus it prevents estrogen from stimulating the receptor. At present, there are no data on its transfer into breastmilk; however, it has been shown to inhibit lactation early postpartum in several studies. In one study, doses of 10-30 mg twice daily early postpartum, completely inhibited postpartum engorgement and lactation. In a second study, tamoxifen doses of 10 mg four times daily significantly reduced serum prolactin and inhibited milk production as well. We do not know the effect of tamoxifen on established milk production. Its prominent effect on reducing prolactin levels will inhibit early lactation and may ultimately inhibit established lactation. Mothers receiving tamoxifen should not breastfeed until we know more about the levels transferred into milk and the plasma/tissue levels found in breastfed infants.

TAMSULOSIN HYDROCHLORIDE; *Flomax, Flomax CR*	L3
Uses: Alpha1 adrenergic antagonist	B
AAP: Not reviewed	
T½= 13 hours; **RID**= ; **Oral** = 90%; **MW**= 445	

Clinical: Although not cleared for women, it is now used for various bladder conditions. No data are available on its transfer to milk. Due to high protein binding and large molecular weight, I anticipate milk levels will be low. But we do not know this for sure at this time.

TAPENTADOL; *Nucynta*	L3
Uses: Opiate analgesic	C
AAP: Not reviewed	
T½= 6 hr; **RID**= ; **Oral** = 32%; **MW**= 257.80	

Clinical: Tapentadol is an opiate analgesic and norepinephrine reuptake inhibitor. There have been no studies done on the effects of tapentadol in breastfeeding mothers. However, from a pharmacokinetic standpoint, we believe it is likely that tapentadol is secreted into breast milk.

TAZAROTENE; *Tazorac*	L3
Uses: Anti-psoriatic	X
AAP: Not reviewed	
T½= 18 hours (met); **RID**= ; **Oral** = Complete; **MW**= 351	

Clinical: Tazarotene is a specialized retinoid for topical use and is used for the topical treatment of stable plaque psoriasis and acne. Only 2-3% of the topically applied drug is absorbed transcutaneously. Little could be detected in the plasma. Data on transmission to breastmilk are not available. The manufacturer reports some is transferred to rodent milk, but it has not been tested in humans.

TEA TREE OIL; *Tea Tree Oil*	L3
Uses: Antibacterial, antifungal	
AAP: Not reviewed	
T½= ; RID= ; Oral = ; MW=	

Clinical: Tee tree oil, as derived from Melaleuca alternifolia, has recently gained popularity for its antiseptic properties. The essential oil, derived by steam distillation of the leaves, contains terpin-4-ol in concentrations of 40% or more. TTO is primarily noted for its antimicrobial effects without irritating sensitive tissues. It is antimicrobial when tested against Candida albicans, E. coli, S. Aureus, Staph. epidermidis, and pseudomonas aeruginosa. In several reports it is suggested to have antifungal properties equivalent to tolnaftate and clotrimazole. Although the use of TTO in adults is mostly nontoxic, the safe use in infants is unknown. Use directly on the nipple should be minimized.

⁹⁹ᴹ TECHNETIUM; *Technetium-99m*	L4
Uses: Radioactive imaging	C
AAP: Radioactive compound that requires temporary cessation of breastfeeding	
T½= <6 hours; RID= ; Oral = Complete; MW=	

Clinical: Radioactive technetium-99M (Tc-99m) is present in milk for at least 15 hours to 3 days, and significant quantities have been reported in the thyroid and gastric mucosa of infants ingesting milk from treated mothers. Technetium is one of the halide elements and is handled, biologically, much like iodine. Like iodine, it concentrates in thyroid tissues, the stomach, and breastmilk of nursing mothers. It has a radioactive half-life of 6.02 hours. In one study using Technetium MAG3 in two mothers receiving 150 MBq of radioactivity, the total percent of ingested radioactivity ranged from 0.7 to 1.6% of the total. These authors suggested that the DTPA salt of technetium would produce the least breastmilk levels and would be preferred in breastfeeding mothers. Use great caution in using radioactive products in breatsfeeding mothers.

TEGASEROD MALEATE; *Zelnorm*	L4
Uses: Treatment of irritable bowel syndrome	B
AAP: Not reviewed	

T½= 11 hours; **RID**= ; **Oral** = 10%; **MW**= 417

Clinical: Tegaserod is a serotonin agonist (stimulant) used to treat the symptoms of irritable bowel syndrome. Oral absorption is only 10 % (fasting) and is reduced 40-65% by food. No data are available on its transfer to human milk. Caution is recommended.

TELBIVUDINE; *Tyzeka*	L4
Uses: Hepatitis B antiviral	B
AAP: Not reviewed	

T½= 40-49 hours; **RID**= ; **Oral** = ; **MW**= 242

Clinical: Telbivudine is a thymidine nucleoside analog that inhibits DNA production. Telbivudine is used in adults with chronic hepatitis B that have evidence of either increased liver function tests or an active infection. It is considered safe in pregnancy, but is very lipid soluble, therefore its transfer into milk may be likely, but probably not clinically relevant. However, this product is intended for chronic use, and exposing an infant to a potential hepatotoxin such as this over a prolonged period is not justified.

TELITHROMYCIN; *Ketek*	L3
Uses: Erythromycin-like antibiotic	C
AAP: Not reviewed	

T½= 9.8 hours; **RID**= ; **Oral** = 57%; **MW**= 812

Clinical: Telithromycin may be useful for more resistant gram-positive infections, particularly pneumococcus, and for anaerobes or H. Influenzae infections. We do not have data on concentrations in milk but they are probably similar to azithromycin or erythromycin, or around 1-3% of the maternal dose. This is not enough to likely cause problems in a breastfeeding infant. One should probably opt for azithromycin until we know more about the milk levels produced by this new drug.   Please be advised that telithromycin is an erythromycin-like antibiotic and perhaps hundreds of drug-drug interactions are possible.

TELMISARTAN; *Micardis, Micardis HCT, Twynsta*	L3
Uses: Angiotensin II receptor antagonist	C

AAP: Not reviewed

T½= 24 hours; **RID**= ; **Oral** = 42-58%; **MW**= 514

Clinical: Telmisartan is a potent antihypertensive. Micardis HCT also contains hydrochlorothiazide 12.5 mg. This agent should never be used in pregnant patients, as fetal demise has been reported with similar agents in this class. No data are available on its use in lactating mothers. However, its use early postpartum in lactating mothers should be approached with caution, particularly in mothers with premature infants.

TEMAZEPAM; *Restoril, PMS-Temazepam*	L3
Uses: Short acting benzodiazepine (Valium-like) hypnotic	X

AAP: Drugs whose effect on nursing infants is unknown but may be of concern

T½= 9.5-12.4 hours; **RID**= ; **Oral** = 90%; **MW**= 301

Clinical: Temazepam is a short acting benzodiazepine that belongs to the Valium family primarily used as a nighttime sedative. In one study levels of temazepam were undetectable in the infants studied although these studies were carried out 15 hours post-dose. Although the study shows low neonatal exposure to temazepam via breastmilk, the infant should be monitored carefully for sleepiness and poor feeding.

TENOFOVIR DISOPROXIL FUMARATE; *Viread*	L3
Uses: Antiretroviral agent	B

AAP: Not reviewed

T½= 17 hours; **RID=** 0.4%; **Oral** = 25-40%; **MW=** 636

Clinical: Tenofovir is used in the management of HIV and hepatitis B infections. It interferes with the viral RNA dependent DNA polymerase, inhibiting viral replication. In monkeys, peak levels in milk were reported to be 0.808 and 0.610 µg/mL. Using this peak data, the relative infant dose would only be 0.4% of the maternal dose. In addition, the oral bioavailability of tenofovir (non salt form) is negligible (5%). Thus the overall risk to a breastfeeding infant would probably be low.

TERAZOSIN HCL; *Hytrin*	L4
Uses: Antihypertensive	C
AAP: Not reviewed	

T½= 9-12 hours; **RID=** ; **Oral** = 90%; **MW=** 423

Clinical: Terazosin is an antihypertensive that belongs to the alpha-1 blocking family. This family is generally very powerful, produces significant orthostatic hypotension and other side effects. Terazosin has rather powerful effects on the prostate and testes producing testicular atrophy in some animal studies (particularly newborn) and is therefore not preferred in pregnant or in lactating women. No data are available on transfer into human milk.

TERBINAFINE; *Lamisil*	L2
Uses: Antifungal	B
AAP: Not reviewed	

T½= 26 hours; **RID=** ; **Oral** = 80%; **MW=** 291

Clinical: Terbinafine is an antifungal agent primarily used for tinea species such as athletes foot and ringworm. Systemic absorption following topical therapy is minimal. In one study, the total excretion of terbinafine in breastmilk ranged from 0.13% to 0.03% of the total maternal dose respectively. Topical absorption through the skin is minimal.

TERBUTALINE; *Bricanyl, Brethine, Bricanyl*	L2
Uses: Bronchodilator for asthma	B
AAP: Maternal medication usually compatible with breastfeeding	

T½= 14 hours; **RID=** 0.2% - 0.3%; **Oral** = 33-50%; **MW=** 225

Clinical: Terbutaline is a popular Beta-2 adrenergic used for bronchodilation in asthmatics. It is secreted into breastmilk but in low quantities. Terbutaline was not detectable in the infant's serum. No untoward effects have been reported in breastfeeding infants.

TERCONAZOLE; *Terazol 3, Terazol 7, Terazol*	L3
Uses: Antifungal, vaginal	C

AAP: Not reviewed

T½= 4-11.3 hours; **RID**= ; **Oral** = Complete; **MW**= 532

Clinical: Terconazole is an antifungal primarily used for vaginal candidiasis. It is similar to fluconazole and itraconazole. At high doses, terconazole is known to enter breastmilk in rodents although no data are available on human milk. The milk levels are probably too small to be clinically relevant.

TERIPARATIDE; *Forteo*	L3
Uses: Human parathyroid hormone	C

AAP: Not reviewed

T½= 1 hour; **RID**= ; **Oral** = Nil; **MW**= 4118

Clinical: Teriparatide is the identical peptide hormone secreted by the parathyroid gland in humans. This leads to an increase in skeletal mass, markers of bone formation and resorption, and bone strength. Teriparatide is used to treat osteoporosis. No studies are available on the levels in breast milk, however, due to the high molecular weight and poor oral bioavailabliltiy, it is unlikely that teriparatide will cross into the milk or be absorbed by an infant.

TETRACYCLINE; *Achromycin, Sumycin, Terramycin,* *Aureomycin, Tetracyn*	L2
Uses: Antibiotic	D

AAP: Maternal medication usually compatible with breastfeeding

T½= 6-12 hours; **RID**= 0.6%-8.44; **Oral** = 75%; **MW**= 444

Clinical: Tetracycline is a broad-spectrum antibiotic with significant side effects in pediatric patients, including dental staining and reduced bone growth. It is secreted into breastmilk in extremely small levels. Because tetracyclines bind to milk calcium they would have reduced oral absorption in the infant. From several studies, the relative infant dose is 0.6%, 4.77% and 8.44%. Thus a high degree of variability exists in these studies. Invariably mixture of tetracyclines in milk would greatly limit their oral bioavailability. The short-term exposure (< 3 weeks) of infants to tetracyclines (via milk) is not contraindicated. However, the long-term exposure of breastfeeding infants to tetracyclines, such as when used daily for acne, could cause problems. The absorption of even small amounts over a prolonged period could result in dental staining.

[201]THALLIUM; *Thallium-[201]*	L3
Uses: Radioactive tracer	X

AAP: Not reviewed

T½= 73 hours; **RID=** ; **Oral =** ; **MW=**

Clinical: Of the several papers in this area, the clinical dose transferred into milk is small. Thallium enters the plasma compartment and is rapidly cleared to other peripheral tissues, thus reported milk levels are quite low. Two sources recommend brief interruptions of 24-96 hours. Thus the interruption of breastfeeding largely depends on the dose and the volume of milk consumed by the infant. Most authors recommend interruption for 24 up to 96 hours, although the NRC commission recommends interruption for 2 weeks.

THEOPHYLLINE; *Aminophylline, Quibron, Theo-Dur, Pulmophylline, Quibron-T/SR*	L3
Uses: Bronchodilator	C

AAP: Maternal medication usually compatible with breastfeeding

T½= 3-12.8 hours; **RID=** 5.9%; **Oral =** 76%; **MW=** 180

Clinical: Theophylline is a methylxanthine bronchodilator. It has a prolonged half-life in neonates which may cause retention. Milk concentrations are approximately equal to the maternal plasma One reported case of irritability and fretful sleeping was reported in an infant exposed to breastmilk only on days when the mother reported taking theophylline. The average milk concentration of theophylline in this case was 0.7 mg/L.

THIABENDAZOLE; *Mintezol*   L3

Uses: Anthelmintic, antiparasitic   C

AAP: Not reviewed

T½= ; **RID=** ; **Oral** = Complete; **MW=** 201

Clinical: Thiabendazole is an antiparasitic agent for the treatment of roundworm, pinworm, hookworm, whipworm, and other parasitic infections. After absorption it is completely eliminated from the plasma by 48 hours although most is excreted by 24 hours. Can be used in children. Although it is effective in pinworms, other agents with less side effects are preferred. No reports on its transfer to breastmilk have been found.

THIAMINE; *Vitamin B1, Betaxin*   L1

Uses: Vitamin

AAP: Maternal medication usually compatible with breastfeeding

T½= ; **RID=** ; **Oral** = Adequate; **MW=** 265

Clinical: Thiamine, also known as Vitamin B-1, is used to treat thiamine deficiency. It is an essential coenzyme in carbohydrate metabolism, combining with adenosine triphosphate to form thiamine pyrophosphate. Thiamine has been shown to cross into human milk, with average concentrations in milk of 200 µg/L under normal circumstances. We do not know what milk levels would be following the use of extraordinarily large oral doses, although it appears that it would be a linear increase in milk levels. Supra-therapeutic doses should be avoided in breastfeeding mothers. Long term high doses (3 gm/day) have been associated with adult toxicity.

THIOPENTAL SODIUM; *Pentothal*   L3

Uses: Barbiturate anesthetic agent   C

AAP: Maternal medication usually compatible with breastfeeding

T½= 3-8 hours; **RID=** 2.6%; **Oral** = Variable; **MW=** 264

Clinical: Thiopental is an ultra short-acting, barbiturate sedative. Used in the induction phase of anesthesia, it rapidly redistributes from the brain to adipose and muscle tissue; hence, the plasma levels are small, and the sedative effects are virtually gone in 20 minutes. Avoid breastfeeding for a few hours.

THIORIDAZINE; *Mellaril, Apo-Thioridazine, Novo-Ridazine*	L4
Uses: Antipsychotic	C

AAP: Not reviewed

T½= 21-24 hours; **RID**= ; **Oral** = Complete; **MW**= 371

Clinical: Thioridazine is a potent phenothiazine tranquilizer. No data are available on its secretion into human milk, but it should be expected to transfer to a limited degree into milk.. Neonatal apnea is associated with this family of drugs.

THIOTHIXENE; *Navane*	L4
Uses: Antipsychotic agent	C

AAP: Not reviewed

T½= 34 hours; **RID**= ; **Oral** = Complete; **MW**= 443

Clinical: Thiothixene is an antipsychotic agent similar in action to the phenothiazines, butyrophenones (Haldol), and chlorprothixene. There are no data on its transfer into human milk. Of this family, thiothixene has a rather higher risk of extrapyramidal symptoms and lowered seizure threshold. These agents generally have long half-lives and some concern exists for long-term exposure. Observe infant for sedation, seizures, or jerks.

THYROTROPIN; *Thyrotropin, TSH, Thyrogen, Thytropar*	L1
Uses: Thyroid-stimulating hormone	C

AAP: Not reviewed

T½= ; **RID**= ; **Oral** = Poor; **MW**= 359

Clinical: Transfer of thyrotropin (TSH) into human milk is negligible and too low to affect a breastfeeding infant. The authors in one study suggest that breastmilk TSH was too low too affect thyroid function in a breastfeeding infant, even with milk from a severe hypothyroid mother.

TIAGABINE; *Gabitril*	L3
Uses: Anticonvulsant	C

AAP: Not reviewed

T½= 7-9 hours; **RID**= ; **Oral** = 90%; **MW**= 412

Clinical: Tiagabine is a GABA inhibitor useful for the treatment of partial epilepsy. No data are available on its transfer to human milk. It has been used in pediatric patients 3-10 years of age. Use in women who are breastfeeding only if the benefits clearly outweigh the risks.

TICARCILLIN; *Ticar, Timentin*	L1
Uses: Penicillin antibiotic	B

AAP: Maternal medication usually compatible with breastfeeding

T½= 0.9-1.3 hours; **RID=** 0.2%; **Oral** = Poor; **MW=** 384

Clinical: Ticarcillin is an extended-spectrum penicillin that is not appreciably absorbed via oral ingestion. In several studies levels in milk were low to trace. Twelve hours after discontinuing ticarcillin, it was undetectable in milk. As with many penicillins, only minimal levels are secreted into milk. Poor oral absorption would limit exposure of breastfeeding infant. May cause changes in GI flora and possibly fungal overgrowth. Timentin is ticarcillin with clavulanate added.

TICLOPIDINE; *Ticlid, Apo-Ticlopidine*	L4
Uses: Inhibits platelet aggregation	B

AAP: Not reviewed

T½= 12.6 hours; **RID=** ; **Oral** = 80%; **MW=** 264

Clinical: Ticlopidine is useful in preventing thromboembolic disorders, increased cardiovascular mortality, stroke, infarcts, and other clotting disorders. Ticlopidine is reported to be excreted into rodent milk. No data are available on penetration into human breastmilk. However it is highly protein bound, and the levels of ticlopidine in plasma are quite low.

TIGECYCLINE; *Tygacil*	L3
Uses: Antibiotic	D

AAP: Not reviewed

T½= 27-42 hours; **RID=** ; **Oral** = Nil; **MW=** 586

Clinical: This is a tetracycline-type antibiotic with potential for staining of teeth. As with the other classic tetracyclines, prolonged exposure (> 3 weeks) is not recommended although brief exposure is probably OK.

TIMOLOL;   *Blocadren, Apo-Timol, Blocadren, Timoptic, Novo-Timol*   L2

Uses: Beta blocker for hypertension and glaucoma   C

AAP: Maternal medication usually compatible with breastfeeding

T½= 4 hours; **RID=** 1.1%; **Oral =** 50%; **MW=** 316

Clinical: Timolol is a beta blocker used for treating hypertension and glaucoma. It is secreted into milk in low levels. Both oral and ophthalmic drops produce modest levels in milk. Untoward effects on infant have not been reported. These levels are probably too small to be clinically relevant.

TINIDAZOLE;   *Tindamax*   L3

Uses: Antimicrobial agent for protozoal and anaerobic bacterial infections   C

AAP: Drugs whose effect on nursing infants is unknown but may be of concern

T½= 11-14.7 hours; **RID=** 12.2%; **Oral =** 100%; **MW=**

Clinical: Tinidazole is an antimicrobial agent that is sometimes used for the treatment of anaerobic infections and protozoal infections such as intestinal amebiasis, Giardia and trichomoniasis. It is similar to metronidazole. Levels in milk are moderate.

TINZAPARIN SODIUM;   *Innohep*   L3

Uses: Anticoagulant low molecular weight heparin   B

AAP: Not reviewed

T½= 3-4 hours; **RID=** ; **Oral =** Nil; **MW=** <7500

Clinical: Tinzaparin is a low molecular weight heparin. The average molecular weight range of tinzaparin is approximately one-half that of regular (unfractionated) heparin (5500-7500 vs 12,000 daltons). No data are available on the transfer of this anticoagulant into human milk but it is likely low. In studies with dalteparin none was found in milk in one study, and only small amounts in another (see dalteparin). In studies with enoxaparin, no changes in anti-Xa activity were noted in breastfed infants. It is very unlikely any would be orally bioavailable.

TIZANIDINE;   *Zanaflex*   L4

Uses: Muscle relaxant   C

AAP: Not reviewed

T½= 13-22 hours; **RID=** ; **Oral** = 40%; **MW=**

Clinical: Tizanidine is a centrally acting muscle relaxant. It has demonstrated efficacy in the treatment of tension headache and spasticity associate with multiple sclerosis. It is not known if it is transferred into human milk although the manufacturer states that due to its lipid solubility, it likely penetrates milk. This product has a long half-life, high lipid solubility, and significant CNS penetration, all factors that would increase milk penetration. While the half-life of the conventional formulation is only 4-8 hours, the half-life of the sustained release formulation is 13-22 hours. Further, 48% of patients complain of sedation. Use caution if used in a breastfeeding mother.

TOBRAMYCIN; *Nebcin, Tobrex, Tobi*	**L3**
Uses: Antibiotic	**D**

AAP: Not reviewed

T½= 2-3 hours; **RID=** 2.6%; **Oral** = Nil; **MW=** 468

Clinical: Levels in milk are low, but could produce minor changes in gut flora. As oral tobramycin is not absorbed orally, systemic levels in infant would be unexpected. Levels in milk are generally low, but could produce minor changes in gut flora. As oral tobramycin is not absorbed orally, systemic levels in infant would be unexpected.

TOCAINIDE; *Tonocard, Xylotocan*	**L4**
Uses: Antiarrhythmic	**C**

AAP: Not reviewed

T½= 11-22 hours; **RID=** 24.5%; **Oral** = 100%; **MW=** 192

Clinical: Reported levels in milk are quite high and it is very well absorbed orally. This product is probably too hazardous to use in a breastfeeding mother. The relative infant dose is high, 24%. Lidocaine would be another choice. Caution is recommended as these levels are quite high and this product is well absorbed.

TOLBUTAMIDE; *Oramide, Orinase, Apo-Tolbutamide, Mobenol, Novo-Butamide*	**L3**
Uses: Antidiabetic	**C**

AAP: Maternal medication usually compatible with breastfeeding

T½= 4.5-6.5 hours; **RID=** 0.02%; **Oral** = Complete; **MW=** 270

Clinical: Tolbutamide is a short-acting sulfonylurea used to stimulate insulin secretion in type II diabetics. Only low levels are secreted into breastmilk. Following a dose of 500 mg twice daily, milk levels in two patients were 3 and 18 µg/L respectively. Maternal serum levels averaged 35 and 45 µg/L. Observe infant closely for jaundice and hypoglycemia.

TOLMETIN SODIUM; *Tolectin*	L3
Uses: Non-steroidal analgesic, used for arthritis, etc.	C
AAP: Maternal medication usually compatible with breastfeeding	
T½= 1-1.5 hours; **RID=** 0.5%; **Oral** = Complete; **MW=** 257	

Clinical: Tolmetin is a standard non-steroidal analgesic. Tolmetin is known to be distributed into milk but in small amounts. The estimate of dose per day an infant would receive is 115 µg/Liter of milk. Tolmetin is sometimes used in pediatric rheumatoid patients (>2 years).

TOLNAFTATE; *Tinactin, Asorbine JR. Antifungal*	L3
Uses: OTC antifungal	
AAP: Not reviewed	
T½= ; **RID=** ; **Oral** = ; **MW=** 307.4090	

Clinical: There are no adequate and well-controlled studies or case reports in breast feeding women. Transcutaneous absorption is minimal. Risk is low.

TOLTERODINE; *Detrol*	L3
Uses: Urinary incontinence	C
AAP: Not reviewed	
T½= 1.9-3.7 hours; **RID=** ; **Oral** = 77%; **MW=**	

Clinical: Tolterodine is a muscarinic anticholinergic agent similar in effect to atropine but is more selective for the urinary bladder. Tolterodine levels in milk have been reported in mice, where offspring exposed to extremely high levels had slightly reduced body weight gain, but no other untoward effects. While it is more selective for the urinary bladder, preclinical trials still showed adverse effects including blurred vision, constipation, and dry mouth in adults. While we have no data on human milk, it is unlikely concentrations will be high enough to produce untoward effects in infants. However, the infant should be monitored for classic anticholinergic symptoms including dry mouth, constipation, poor tearing, etc.

TOPIRAMATE; *Topamax*	L3
Uses: Anticonvulsant	C
AAP: Not reviewed	

T½= 18-24 hours; **RID=** 24.5%; **Oral =** 75%; **MW=** 339

Clinical: Topiramate may be used during breastfeeding with close monitoring. The amount transferred into milk is relatively high, however there have been no reports of adverse effects in the breastfed infant. Plasma levels in two infant were 10-20% of maternal plasma levels. Topiramate has become increasingly popular due to its fewer adverse side effects. Due to the fact that the plasma levels found in breastfeeding infants were significantly less than in maternal plasma, the risk of using this product in breastfeeding mothers is probably acceptable. Close observation for sedation is advised.

TORSEMIDE; *Demadex*	L3
Uses: Potent Loop diuretic	B
AAP: Not reviewed	

T½= 3.5 hours; **RID=** ; **Oral =** 80%; **MW=** 348

Clinical: Torsemide is a potent loop diuretic generally used in congestive heart failure and other conditions which require a strong diuretic. There are no reports of its transfer into human milk. Its extraordinary high protein binding would likely limit its transfer into human milk. As with many diuretics, reduction of plasma volume and hypotension may adversely reduce milk production although this is rare. See furosemide.

TOXOPLAMOSIS	L3
Uses: Infectious disease	

AAP: Not reviewed

T½= ; **RID=** ; **Oral =** ; **MW=**

Clinical: According to the CDC, there are no studies documenting breast milk transmission of toxoplasma in humans.

TRAMADOL AND ACETAMINOPHEN; *Ultracet*	L2
Uses: Analgesic	C

AAP: Not reviewed

T½= ; **RID=** ; **Oral =** ; **MW=**

Clinical: Ultracet is the combination of 37.5 mg of tramadol (Ultram) and 325 mg acetaminophen. See individual monographs.

TRAMADOL; *Ultram*	L2
Uses: Analgesic	C

AAP: Not reviewed

T½= 7 hours; **RID=** 2.9%; **Oral =** 60%; **MW=** 263

Clinical: New data seem to suggest that transfer into milk is low. No infant neurobehaviroal effects were noted in one good study. In a recent study of 75 mothers who received 100 mg every 6 hours after Caesarian section, milk samples were taken on days 2-4 postpartum in transitional milk. The relative infant dose was 2.24% and 0.64% for rac-tramadol and its desmethyl metabolite, respectively. No significant neurobehavioral adverse effects were noted between controls and exposed infants.

TRAZODONE; *Desyrel, Oleptro, Trazorel, Apo-Trazodone, Novo-Trazodone*	L2
Uses: Antidepressant, serotonin reuptake inhibitor	C

AAP: Drugs whose effect on nursing infants is unknown but may be of concern

T½= 4-9 hours; **RID=** 2.8%; **Oral =** 65%; **MW=** 372

Clinical: Trazodone is an antidepressant whose structure is dissimilar to the tricyclics and to the other antidepressants. On a weight basis, an adult would receive 0.77 mg/kg whereas a breastfeeding infant, using this data, would consume only 0.005 mg/kg. The authors estimate that about 0.6% of the maternal dose was ingested by the infant over 24 hours.

TRETINOIN; *Retin - A, Renova, Stieva-A, Vitamin A Acid*	L3
Uses: Treatment of acne	C
AAP: Not reviewed	
$T\frac{1}{2}$= 2 hours; **RID=** ; **Oral** = 70%; **MW**= 300	

Clinical: Topical application is hardly even absorbed transcutaneously. However, it should never be administered ORALLY to breastfeeding mothers.

TRIAMCINOLONE ACETONIDE; *Nasacort, Azmacort, Tri-Nasal, Aristocort, Azmacort, Kenalog, Triaderm*	L3
Uses: Corticosteroid	C
AAP: Not reviewed	
$T\frac{1}{2}$= 88 minutes; **RID=** ; **Oral** = Complete; **MW**= 434	

Clinical: Triamcinolone is a typical corticosteroid (see prednisone) that is available for topical, intranasal, injection, inhalation, and oral use. When applied topically to the nose (Nasacort) or to the lungs (Azmacort), only minimal doses are used and plasma levels are exceedingly low to undetectable. Although no data are available on triamcinolone secretion into human milk, it is likely that the milk levels would be exceedingly low and not clinically relevant when administered via inhalation or intranasally. While the oral adult dose is 4-48 mg/day, the inhaled dose is 200 µg three times daily, and the intranasal dose is 220 µg/day. There is virtually no risk to the infant following use of the intranasal products in breastfeeding mothers.

TRIAMTERENE; *Dyrenium*	L3
Uses: Diuretic	C
AAP: Not reviewed	
$T\frac{1}{2}$= 1.5-2.5 hours; **RID=** ; **Oral** = 30-70%; **MW**= 253	

Clinical: Triamterene is a potassium-sparing diuretic, commonly used in combination with thiazide diuretics such as hydrochlorothiazide (Dyazide). Plasma levels average 26-30 nanograms/mL. No data are available on the transfer of triamterene into human milk, but it is known to transfer into animal milk. Because of the availability of other less dangerous diuretics, triamterene should be used as a last resort in breastfeeding mothers.

TRIAZOLAM; *Halcion, Apo-Triazo, Novo-Triolam*	L3
Uses: Benzodiazepine (Valium-like) hypnotic	X
AAP: Not reviewed	

T½= 1.5-5.5 hours; **RID=** ; **Oral** = 85%; **MW=** 343

Clinical: Triazolam is a typical benzodiazepine used as a nighttime sedative. Animal studies indicate that triazolam is secreted into milk although levels in human milk have not been reported. As with all the benzodiazepines, some penetration into breastmilk is likely.

TRICLOSAN; *Adacept, Ameriwash*	L3
Uses: Antibacterial, antifungal	
AAP: Not reviewed	

T½= ; **RID=** ; **Oral** = ; **MW=** 289.5

Clinical: In a study including 36 mothers, investigators reported finding triclosan in all of the breastmilk samples. However triclosan is overty toxic, although its use is not recommended in pregnant and breastfeeding mothers.

TRIMEBUTINE MALEATE; *Apo-Trimebutine, Modulon*	L3
Uses: 5HT3 receptor antagonist	
AAP: Not reviewed	

T½= 10-12 hours; **RID=** 0%; **Oral** = ; **MW=** 387

Clinical: Trimebutine is used to treat irritable bowel syndrome and to accelerate intestinal transit following abdominal surgery. Trimebutine maleate is not available in the U.S. No data are available on the use of this product in breastfeeding mothers.

TRIMEPRAZINE; *Temaril, Panectyl*	L3
Uses: Antihistamine, antipruritic	C
AAP: Not reviewed	
T½= 5 hours; **RID=** ; **Oral** = 70%; **MW=** 298	
Clinical: Trimeprazine is an antihistamine from the phenothiazine family used for itching. It is secreted into human milk but in very low levels. Exact data is not available.	

TRIMETHOBENZAMIDE; *Tigan, Trimazide, Tebamide, T-Gen, Arrestin, Ticon*	L4
Uses: Antiemetic, antivertigo	C
AAP: Not reviewed	
T½= Short; **RID=** ; **Oral** = Good; **MW=**	
Clinical: Trimethobenzamide is an older generation antiemetics whose use has been supplanted by newer more effective agents. It is most commonly used in suppository form in adults and rarely in infants. No data are available on breastmilk levels. It is unlikely the amount of trimethobenzamide present in breastmilk would produce a clinical effect in an infant.	

TRIMETHOPRIM; *Proloprim, Trimpex*	L2
Uses: Antibiotic	C
AAP: Maternal medication usually compatible with breastfeeding	
T½= 8-10 hours; **RID=** 9%; **Oral** = Complete; **MW=** 290	
Clinical: Long-term use of trimethoprim during breastfeeding should be avoided. Otherwise trimethoprim is commonly used in full-term or older infants (>1 week old) with no untoward effects. Because it may interfere with folate metabolism, its long-term use should be avoided in breastfeeding mothers, or the infant should be supplemented with folic acid. However, trimethoprim apparently poses few problems in full term or older infants where it is commonly used clinically.	

TRIPELENNAMINE; *PBZ, Colrex, Tromide, Pyrabenzamine*	L4
Uses: Antihistamine	B
AAP: Not reviewed	
T½= 2-3 hours; **RID=** ; **Oral** = Complete; **MW=** 255	

Clinical: Tripelennamine is an older class of antihistamine. This product is generally not recommended in pediatric patients, particularly neonates due to increased sleep apnea. The drug has been shown to be secreted into milk of animals. No human data exist. Alternatives include: loratadine, cetirizine, or fexofenadrine.

TRIPROLIDINE; *Actidil, Actacin, Actifed*	L1
Uses: Antihistamine	C

AAP: Maternal medication usually compatible with breastfeeding

T½= 5 hours; **RID=** 1.8%; **Oral** = Complete; **MW=** 278

Clinical: Triprolidine is an antihistamine. It is secreted into milk but in very small levels and is marketed with pseudoephedrine as Actifed. The relative infant dose is less than 1.8% of the weight-normalized maternal dose. This dose is far too low to be clinically relevant.

TRIPTORELIN PAMOATE; *Trelstar LA, Trelstar Depo, Trelstar*	L3
Uses: Analog of luteinizing hormone releasing hormone	X

AAP: Not reviewed

T½= 3 hour IV; **RID=** ; **Oral** = Nil; **MW=** 1699

Clinical: It is unlikely this agent would penetrate milk due to its high molecular weight. Also, it is not orally bioavailable, so it is very unlikely to harm a breastfeeding infant. Continuous use in breastfeeding mothers would ultimately lead to reduced levels of ovulation and sex steroids. Thus it is difficult to discern what if any effect this agent would have on milk production in breastfeeding mothers. Continuous use in breastfeeding mothers would ultimately lead to reduced levels of ovulation and sex steroids. In a study in males, prolactin levels were actually increased. Thus it is difficult to discern what if any effect this agent would have on milk production in breastfeeding mothers. Some caution is recommended until more is known about this drugs effect on milk production. It is extremely unlikely this agent would penetrate milk due to its high molecular weight. Also, it is not orally bioavailable, so it is very unlikely to harm a breastfeeding infant.

TROPICAMIDE; *Mydral, Mydriacyl, Tropicacyl, Diotrope*	L3
Uses: Mydriatic ophthalmic agent	C
AAP: Not reviewed	
T½= ; **RID=** ; **Oral =** ; **MW=** 284	

Clinical: Tropicamide is used as a short-acting pupil dilator used in diagnostic procedures. It is an antimuscarinic agent which produces competitive antagonism of the actions of acetylcholine, thus preventing the sphincter muscle of the iris and the muscle of the ciliary body from responding to cholinergic stimulation. It is unlikely that systemic levels in adults will be sufficient to produce clinically relevant levels in milk. Infants, however should be observed for anticholinergic effects (dry mouth, mydriasis, sedation, tachycardia). A brief waiting period of 3-4 hours would eliminate most risks.

TUBERCULIN PURIFIED PROTEIN DERIVATIVE; *Tubersol, Aplisol, Sclavo, PPD, Mantoux*	L2
Uses: Tuberculin skin test	C
AAP: Not reviewed	
T½= ; **RID=** ; **Oral =** ; **MW=**	

Clinical: TB tests are generally safe to have during breastfeeding. It is a one-time test with minimal risks associated with administration. It is composed of proteins, which are unlikely to enter breast milk. Adverse effects are usually local.

TYPHOID VACCINE; *Vivotif Berna, Typhim Vi*	L3
Uses: Vaccination	C
AAP: Not reviewed	
T½= ; **RID=** ; **Oral =** ; **MW=**	

Clinical: Typhoid vaccine promotes active immunity to typhoid fever. It is available in an oral form (Ty21a) which is a live attenuated vaccine for oral administration. The parenteral (injectable) form is derived from acetone-treated killed and dried bacteria, phenol-inactive bacteria, or a special capsular polysaccharide vaccine extracted from killed S. typhi Ty21a strains. No data are available on its transfer into human milk. If immunization is required, a killed species would be preferred, as infection of the neonate would be unlikely.

ULIPRISTAL ACETATE; *Ella*	L3
Uses: Progesterone agonist/antagonist	X
AAP: Not reviewed	
T½= ; **RID=** ; **Oral** = 100%; **MW=** 475.6	

Clinical: Ella is a selective progesterone receptor modulator used for emergency contraception within 120 hours of unprotected sex. No data are available, but since it is a steroid, it is unlikely to enter milk readily.

URSODIOL; *Actigall, Urso*	L3
Uses: Bile acid for dissolving gall stones	B
AAP: Not reviewed	
T½= ; **RID=** ; **Oral** = 90%; **MW=** 392	

Clinical: Ursodiol (ursodeoxycholic acid) is a bile salt found in small amounts in humans that is used to dissolve cholesterol gallstones. It is almost completely absorbed orally via the portal circulation and is extracted almost completely by the liver. Only trace amounts are found in the plasma and it is not likely significant amounts would be present in milk. While no breastfeeding data are available, only small amounts of bile salts are known to be present in milk. It is not likely with the low levels of ursodiol in the maternal plasma, that clinically relevant amounts would enter milk.

VALACYCLOVIR; *Valtrex*	L1
Uses: Antiviral, for herpes simplex	B
AAP: Not reviewed	
T½= 2.5-3 hours; **RID=** 4.7%; **Oral** = 54%; **MW=**	

Clinical: Valacyclovir is rapidly metabolized to acyclovir whjch transfers to human milk. However, the levels in milk are miniscule compared to the clinical doses administered directly to infants. Acyclovir is quite safe for infants with few reported risks or side effects. The risks to a breastfeeding infants would be minimal.   The amount of acyclovir in breast milk after valacyclovir administration is considerably less than that used in therapeutic dosing of neonates.

VALERIAN OFFICINALIS; *Valerian Root*	L3
Uses: Herbal sedative	
AAP: Not reviewed	

T½= ; **RID=** ; **Oral =** ; **MW=**

Clinical: Valerian root is most commonly used as a sedative/hypnotic. Of the numerous chemicals present in the root, the most important chemical group appears to be the valepotriates. This family consists of at least a dozen or more related compounds and is believed responsible for the sedative potential of this plant although it is controversial. The combination of numerous components may inevitability account for the sedative response. Controlled studies in man have indicated a sedative/hypnotic effect with fewer night awakenings and significant somnolence. The toxicity of valerian root appears to be low, with only minor side effects reported. However, the valepotriates have been found to be cytotoxic, with alkylating activity similar to other nitrogen mustard-like anticancer agents. Should this prove to be so in vivo, it may preclude the use of this product in humans. No data are available on the transfer of valerian root compounds into human milk. However, the use of sedatives in breastfeeding mothers is generally discouraged, due to a possible increased risk of SIDS.

VALGANCICLOVIR; *Valcyte, Cytovene*	L3
Uses: Antiviral	C
AAP: Not reviewed	

T½= 4 hours; **RID=** ; **Oral =** 61%; **MW=** 390

Clinical: Valganciclovir is a prodrug that is rapidly metabolized to the active antiviral drug ganciclovir. It is used for cytomegalovirus infections particularly in HIV infected patients. The oral bioavailability of valganciclovir is 60% while only 6% with its active metabolite ganciclovir. Further it is very water soluble and lipophobic, which would suggest milk levels will be low. No data are available on its use in breastfeeding mothers but its oral absorption in the infant is likely low.

VALPROIC ACID; *Depakene, Depakote, Stavzor, Novo-Valproic, Deproic*	L2
Uses: Anticonvulsant	D
AAP: Maternal medication usually compatible with breastfeeding	

T½= 14 hours; **RID=** 1.4% - 1.7%; **Oral =** Complete; **MW=** 144

Clinical: Valproic acid usage during breastfeeding is probably safe. The levels of valproic acid secreted into milk are minimal, and pose little risk to the breastfed infant. Monitor the infant for changes in platelet levels and liver enzymes. Most authors agree that the amount of valproic acid transferring to the infant via milk is low. Breastfeeding would appear safe. However, the infant may need monitoring for liver and platelet changes.

VALSARTAN; *Diovan, Valturna*	L3
Uses: Antihypertensive	C
AAP: Not reviewed	
T½= 9 hours; **RID**= ; **Oral** = 23%; **MW**=	

Clinical: Valsartan is a new angiotensin II receptor antagonist used to treat hypertension. While it is believed to enter the milk of rodents, no human data are available.[1,2] Use with caution in breastfeeding mothers.

VANCOMYCIN; *Vancocin*	L1
Uses: Antibiotic	C
AAP: Not reviewed	
T½= 5.6 hours; **RID**= 6.7%; **Oral** = Minimal; **MW**= 1449	

Clinical: Vancomycin is probably safe to use during breastfeeding. Transfer to milk is minimal since it is a relatively large molecule, and oral absorption is poor. Possible side effect is diarrhea although there have been no reports of harm to the breastfed infant.

VARENICLINE; *Chantix*	L4
Uses: Smoking cessation	C
AAP: Not reviewed	
T½= 24 hours; **RID**= ; **Oral** = High; **MW**= 361	

Clinical: Varenicline is used to assist smoking cessation. There have been no studies performed on the transfer of varenicline into human milk, but it is nearly identical in structure to nicotine and would probably transfer into human milk easily. Caution should be used in breastfeeding mothers.

VARICELLA ZOSTER VACCINE; *Varivax*	L2
Uses: Vaccination for varicella (chickenpox)	C

AAP: Not reviewed

T½= ;   **RID=** 0%;   **Oral =** ;   **MW=**

Clinical: A live attenuated varicella vaccine (Varivax - Merck) was recently approved for marketing by the US Food and Drug Administration. The Oka/Merck strain used in the vaccine is attenuated by passage in human and embryonic guinea pig cell cultures. It is not known if the vaccine-acquired VZV is secreted in human milk, nor its infectiousness to infants. Interestingly, in two women with varicella-zoster infections, the virus was not culturable from milk. Mothers of immunodeficient infants should not breastfeed following use of this vaccine. Recommendations for Use: Varicella vaccine is only recommended for children >1 year of age up to 12 years of age with no history of varicella infection. Both the AAP and the Center for Disease Control approve the use of varicella-zoster vaccines in breastfeeding mothers, if the risk of infection is high.

VARICELLA-ZOSTER VIRUS; *Chickenpox*	L4
Uses: Chickenpox	

AAP: Not reviewed

T½= ;   **RID=** ;   **Oral =** ;   **MW=**

Clinical: Chickenpox virus has been reported to be transferred via breastmilk in one 27 year old mother who developed chickenpox postpartum. Her 2 month old son also developed the disease 16 days after mother. Chickenpox virus was detected in the mother's milk and may suggest that transmission can occur via breastmilk. However, in a study of 2 breastfeeding patients who developed varicella-herpes zoster infections, in neither case was the virus isolated and cultured from their milk. According to the American Academy of Pediatrics, neonates born to mothers with active varicella should be placed in isolation at birth and, if still hospitalized, until 21 or 28 days of age, depending on whether they received VZIG (Varicella Zoster Immune Globulin). Candidates for VZIG include: immunocompromised children, pregnant women, and a newborn infant whose mother has onset of VZV within 5 days before or 48 hours after delivery.

VASOPRESSIN; *Pitressin, Pressyn*	L3
Uses: Antidiuretic hormone	C

AAP: Not reviewed

T½= 10-20 minutes;   **RID=** ;   **Oral =** None;   **MW=**

Clinical: Vasopressin, also know as the antidiuretic hormone, is a small peptide (8 amino acids) that is normally secreted by the posterior pituitary. It reduces urine production by the kidney. Although it probably passes to some degree into human milk, it is rapidly destroyed in the GI tract by trypsin and must be administered by injection or intranasally. Hence, oral absorption by a nursing infant is very unlikely. Desmopressin is virtually identical and milk levels have been reported to be very low. See desmopressin.

VENLAFAXINE; *Effexor*	L3
Uses: Antidepressant	C
AAP: Not reviewed	

T½= 5 hours (venlafaxine); **RID=** 6.8% - 8.1%; **Oral =** 92%; **MW=** 313

Clinical: The clinical dose of venlafaxine transferred via milk is about 6.4% for both metabolite and parent drug. Thus far, no reports of adverse effects have been found following exposure via milk. However, recent data has suggested that infants exposed in utero, may have profound adverse effects immediately upon delivery. These include: respiratory distress, cyanosis, apnea, seizures, temperature instability, etc. It is not known if these adverse events are due to a direct toxic effect of venlafaxine on the fetus, or due to a discontinuation (withdrawal) syndrome. To avoid this complication, patients may need to be withdrawn carefully over a prolonged period prior to delivery. This should only be done under close observation however.

VERAPAMIL; *Calan, Isoptin, Covera-HS, Apo-Verap, Novo-Veramil*	L2
Uses: Calcium channel blocker for hypertension	C
AAP: Maternal medication usually compatible with breastfeeding	

T½= 3-7 hours; **RID=** 0.2%; **Oral =** 90%; **MW=** 455

Clinical: Verapamil is a typical calcium channel blocker used as an antihypertensive. It is secreted into milk but in very low levels, which are highly controversial. From several studies, the relative infant dose would vary from 0.15%, 0.98%, and 0.18%. Regardless of the variability, the relative amount transferred to the infant is still quite small.

VERTEPORFIN; *Visudyne*	**L3**
Uses: Photosensitizing agent to treat macular degeneration	**C**

AAP: Not reviewed

T½= 5-6 hours;   **RID=** ;   **Oral** = Nil;   **MW=** 718

Clinical: Verteporfin is a photosensitizing agent, that produces significant but brief plasma and milk levels. It is unlikely that present in milk would be orally absorbed however. But due to the risks of this medication, breast milk should be pumped and discarded for 24 hours.   The manufacturer reports verteporfin and its metabolites have been found in the breast milk of one women after a 6 mg/m^2 infusion.   Milk levels were up to 66% of the corresponding plasma levels. Verteporfin was undetectable after 12 hours but its metabolites were present for up to 48 hours. A waiting period of 24 hours is recommended.

VIGABATRIN; *Sabril*	**L3**
Uses: Anticonvulsant	**C**

AAP: Not reviewed

T½= 7 hours;   **RID=** ;   **Oral** = 50%;   **MW=** 129

Clinical: Vigabatrin is a newer anticonvulsant. It is an effective adjunctive anticonvulsant for the treatment of multi-drug resistant complex partial seizures. It has also shown efficacy in controlling seizures and spasm in infants 3 months and older. No data are available on its transfer into human milk.   Some caution is recommended in breastfeeding mothers.

VITAMIN A; *Aquasol A, Del-VI-A, Vitamin A, Retinol*	**L3**
Uses: Vitamin supplement	**A**

AAP: Not reviewed

T½= ;   **RID=** ;   **Oral** = Complete;   **MW=** 286

Clinical: Be cautious of overdose. High doses of vitamin will surely end up in milk and could produce toxic sequelae in breastfed infants if doses are high and chronic. Be cautious and do not use supratherapeutic doses in breastfeeding mothers. Chronic exposure to levels of 4,000 IU/kg daily for 6 or more months could be hazardous. Liver damage can occur at doses as low as 15,000 IU per day. In infants, a bulging fontanel is also indicative of Vitamin A toxicity. At this point we do not know if vitamin A levels in milk correlate with maternal plasma levels, but they probably do. Caution is recommended in supratherapeutic dosing in breastfeeding mothers.

VITAMIN B-12; *Cyanocobalamin, Rubramin*	L1
Uses: Vitamin supplement	A

AAP: Maternal medication usually compatible with breastfeeding

T½= ; **RID=** ; **Oral** = Variable; **MW=** 1355

Clinical: B12 deficiency states are extremely hazardous to a fetus or a breastfeeding infant. Breastfeeding mothers who are vegans or even vegetarians should probably be supplemented with B12 in some form.

VITAMIN D; *Calciferol, Delta-D, Vitamin D, Calcijex, Drisdol, Hytakerol*	L2
Uses: Vitamin D supplement	A

AAP: Maternal medication usually compatible with breastfeeding

T½= ; **RID=** ; **Oral** = Variable; **MW=** 396

Clinical: The amount of vitamin D in milk is quite low, and rickets has been increasingly noted in the breastfeeding infant. The AAP presently recommends the use of 200 IU/day in breastfeeding infants. New data now suggests that supplementing the mother with 2000-4000 IU/day vitamin D can increase levels in milk and the plasma compartment of the infant. However, these levels still may not provide the daily allowance of 200-400 IU/day.

VITAMIN E; *Alpha Tocopherol, Aquasol E*	L2
Uses: Vitamin E supplement	A

AAP: Not reviewed

T½= 282 hours (IV); **RID=** ; **Oral** = Variable; **MW=** 431

Clinical: Vitamin E is a fat soluble vitamin. Levels in milk are moderately low and seem relatively insensitive to supplementation until the maternal dose is quite high (thousands of units). Vitamin E levels seem to trend downward with each week of lactation. Premature infants have higher requirements for vitamin E and supplementation of the mother while breastfeeding a premature infant may be useful. However, a number of infant deaths years ago clearly show that high levels can be hazardous. The application of concentrated vitamin E directly on the nipple could be hazardous and should be avoided, although less concentrated forms (50-100 IU) are probably safe.

WARFARIN; *Coumadin, Panwarfin, Warfilone*	L2
Uses: Anticoagulant	X

AAP: Maternal medication usually compatible with breastfeeding

T½= 1-2.5 days; **RID=** ; **Oral =** Complete; **MW=** 308

Clinical: Warfarin usage during breastfeeding is probably safe. There have been no reports of adverse effects, although observe for bruising or bleeding in the breastfed infant. To counteract the effects of high-dose warfarin, Vitamin K supplementation may be given to premature infants. According to the authors of several studies, maternal warfarin apparently poses little risk to a nursing infant and thus far has not produced bleeding anomalies in breastfed infants. Observe infant for bleeding such as excessive bruising or reddish petechia (spots). While the risks in breastfeeding premature infants (which are more susceptible to intracranial bleeding) is still low, oral supplementation with vitamin K1 will preclude any chance of hemorrhage. Even modest doses of Vitamin K1 counteract high doses of warfarin.

WEST NILE FEVER;	L4
Uses: Viral febrile infection	

AAP: Not reviewed

T½= ; **RID=** ; **Oral =** ; **MW=**

Clinical: Thus far, there has been no documented occurrence of a mother passing the West Nile virus via maternal milk. Infected mosquitoes are the primary vector for West Nile virus although both hard and soft ticks have been found infected with West Nile virus in nature, but their role in the transmission and maintenance of the virus is uncertain. Mosquitoes, largely bird-feeding species, are the principal vectors of West Nile virus. For answers to questions about West Nile virus, please see the CDC web site.

YELLOW FEVER VACCINE; *YF-Vax, Arilvax, Stamaril*	L4
Uses: Vaccine	C
AAP: Not reviewed	

T½= ; **RID**= 0%; **Oral** = ; **MW**=

Clinical: The CDC recommends that due to certain risks that breastfeeding mothers not be immunized unless they are entering regions of high risk. This vaccine is a live attenuated vaccine, so there is significant risk the infant will at least ingest some virus. A recent report strongly suggests that the yellow fever virus (17DD) may be transmitted via milk. Because of the risk for viral encephalitis, in no instance should infants aged <6 months receive yellow fever vaccine. Therefore, if the infant is between 1 and 5 months, the mother should NOT be immunized. If the infant is >6 months, and the mother is entering a region of high risk for the infection, then at least the mother, and perhaps the infant should be immunized directly. Based on a theoretic risk of transmission via milk, the CDC now strongly recommends against the use of yellow fever vaccines in breastfeeding mothers, except in situations where the risk of contracting the disease is unavoidable. Check the CDC for current recommendations. In those mothers who received the yellow fever vaccine, studies found that maternal levels of 17D virus are no longer present in maternal serum after 13 days. This would suggest that the risk to a breastfed infant 13 days after immunization is low to nil.

ZAFIRLUKAST; *Accolate*	L3
Uses: Leukotriene inhibitor for Asthma	B
AAP: Not reviewed	

T½= 10-13 hours; **RID**= 0.7%; **Oral** = Poor; **MW**= 575

Clinical: Zafirlukast levels in milk are low. Zafirlukast is poorly absorbed when administered with food. It is likely the oral absorption via ingestion of breastmilk would be low. The manufacturer recommends against using in breastfeeding mothers.

ZALEPLON; *Sonata, Starnoc*	L2
Uses: Hypnotic agent used for insomnia	C
AAP: Not reviewed	

T½= 1.2 hours; **RID=** 1.5%; **Oral =** Complete; **MW=** 305

Clinical: Zaleplon is a nonbenzodiazepine hypnotic sedative that interacts at the GABA receptor. Milk levels are low and decreased rapidly following a peak at 1.2 hours to less than 3 µg/L four hours following administration. The authors suggest that these levels would be subclinical to the infant.

ZIDOVUDINE; *Retrovir, Combivir, Novo-Azt*	L3
Uses: Antiretroviral agent used in HIV	C
AAP: Not reviewed	

T½= <3 hours; **RID=** 0.4%; **Oral =** 61%; **MW=** 267

Clinical: Milk levels are approximately 3.21 times higher than the maternal serum, although zidovudine has a rather brief half-life. However infant serum levels are still supratherapeutic (2.5 fold the maternal serum level) which is somewhat inexplicable. In adults, and apparently infants, zidovudine has a delayed terminal phase half-life (4.8 hours) longer than its initial half-life (<3 hours). The rather high serum levels in infant is worrisome and some caution is recommended although no untoward effects were reported in this study of 18 patients. Close monitoring of the infant for changes in CBC (granulocytopenia, anemia, leukopenia), liver function, CNS symptoms (i.e. headache, seizures), drug-induced myopathy, and numerous other symptoms, is recommended.

ZILEUTON; *Zyflo*	L3
Uses: Lipoxygenase inhibitor	C
AAP: Not reviewed	

T½= 2.5 hours; **RID=** ; **Oral =** ; **MW=** 236

Clinical: Zileuton is used for chronic treatment of asthma. It inhibits leukotriene formation, which in turn minimizes inflammation and bronchoconstriction in the airways. No data are available on its transfer into human milk. It is not significantly toxic nor does it have severe side effects.

ZINC SALTS; *Zinc*	L2
Uses: Zinc supplements	
AAP: Not reviewed	
$T\frac{1}{2}$= ; **RID**= ; **Oral** = 41%; **MW**=	

Clinical: Zinc is an essential element that is required for enzymatic function within the cell. Zinc deficiencies have been documented in newborns and premature infants with symptoms such as anorexia nervosa, arthritis, diarrheas, eczema, recurrent infections, and recalcitrant skin problems. The Recommended Daily Allowance for adults is 12-15 mg/day. The average oral dose of supplements is 25-50 mg/day; higher doses may lead to gastritis. Excessive intake is hazardous. Zinc absorption by the infant from human milk is high, averaging 41%, which is significantly higher than from soy or cow formulas (14% and 31% respectively). Minimum daily requirements of zinc in full term infants vary from 0.3 to 0.5 mg/kg/day. Daily ingestion of zinc from breastmilk has been estimated to be 0.35 mg/kg/day and declines over the first 17 weeks of life as older neonates require less zinc due to slower growth rate. Supplementation with 25-50 mg/day is probably safe, but excessive doses are discouraged. Another author has shown that zinc levels in breastmilk are independent of maternal plasma zinc concentrations or dietary zinc intake. Other body pools of zinc (i.e., liver and bone) are perhaps the source of zinc in breastmilk. Therefore, higher levels of oral zinc intake probably have minimal effect on zinc concentrations in milk but excessive doses are not recommended.

ZIPRASIDONE; *Geodon*	L2
Uses: Antipsychotic	C
AAP: Not reviewed	
$T\frac{1}{2}$= 7 hours; **RID**= 0.07% - 1.2%; **Oral** = 60%; **MW**= 419	

Clinical: Transfer of ziprasidone into milk appears to be minimal, although our data is only from case reports. Ziprasidone usage during breastfeeding is probably safe. Quetiapine is a suitable alternative in the same drug class. Observe for sedation in the breastfed infant. No adverse effects have been reported in the infant.

ZOLMITRIPTAN; *Zomig, Zomig-ZMT, Rapimelt*	L3
Uses: Migraine analgesic	C
AAP: Not reviewed	
T½= 3 hours; **RID=** ; **Oral =** 48%; **MW=**	

Clinical: Zolmitriptan is specifically indicated for treating acute migraine headaches. Zolmitriptan is structurally similar to sumatriptan but has better oral bioavailability, higher penetration into the CNS, and may have dual mechanisms of action. No data are available on its penetration into human milk. See sumatriptan as preferred alternate.

ZOLPIDEM TARTRATE; *Ambien, Ambien CR, Edluar*	L3
Uses: Sedative, sleep aid	C
AAP: Maternal medication usually compatible with breastfeeding	
T½= 2.5-5 hours; **RID=** 4.7% - 19.1%; **Oral =** 70%; **MW=** 307	

Clinical: Zolpidem transfer to milk is variable but moderately high. It is probably okay to use during breastfeeding. One case of infant sedation and poor appetite related to zolpidem use has been reported following the nightly use of sertraline (100mg) and 10 mg Zolpidem. Use of sedatives in breastfeeding mothers is of some concern, particularly those with premature or young neonates, and those with weak infants. This drug should be avoided in mothers with infants subject to apnea. Zopiclone or eszopiclone are preferred sedatives in breastfeeding.

ZONISAMIDE; *Zonegran*	L5
Uses: Anti-convulsant	C
AAP: Not reviewed	
T½= 63 hours; **RID=** 33.3%; **Oral =** ; **MW=** 212	

Clinical: Zonisamide is a broad-spectrum anticonvulsant medication chemically classified as a sulfonamide. In one study, using the highest reported milk level, the relative infant dose would be 33% of the maternal dose. This is quite high. Significant caution is recommended with this medication as a number of pediatric adverse effects have been noted in older children.

ZOPICLONE; *Apo-Zopiclone, Dom-Zopiclone, PMS-Zopiclone, Rhovan, Alti-Zopiclone, Ratio-Zopiclone*	L2
Uses: Hypnotic sedative	C
AAP: Not reviewed	

T½= 4-5 hours; **RID=** 1.5%; **Oral** = 75%; **MW=** 388

Clinical: Use of sedatives in breastfeeding mothers is of some concern, particularly those with premature or young neonates, and those with weak infants. This drug should be avoided in mothers with infants subject to apnea. Zopiclone is the preferred choice for sedatives during breastfeeding.

ZUCLOPENTHIXOL; *Clopixol-Acuphase, Clopixol Depot, Clopixol*	L3
Uses: Antipsychotic agent	C
AAP: Not reviewed	

T½= 20 hours; **RID=** 0.4% - 0.9%; **Oral** = 49%; **MW=** 443-555

Clinical: Reported levels in milk are low as are the reported relative infant doses. The plasma levels of zuclopenthixol in infants were low in both studies. No untoward effects were noted in the infants although some caution is recommended with prolonged exposure to this medication.

Index

Note: Drug names in ALL CAPS indicate generic drug name.